100 Questions & Answers About Multiple Sclerosis

William A. Sheremata, MD, FRCPC, FACP

Professor of Neurology
University of Miami
School of Medicine
and
Bob Hope Parkinson Research Center

JONES AND BARTLETT PUBLISHERS
Sudbury, Massachusetts
BOSTON   TORONTO   LONDON   SINGAPORE

World Headquarters

Jones and Bartlett Publishers	Jones and Bartlett Publishers Canada	Jones and Bartlett Publishers International
40 Tall Pine Drive	6339 Ormindale Road	Barb House, Barb Mews
Sudbury, MA 01776	Mississauga, ON L5V	London W6 7PA
978-443-5000	1J2	UK
info@jbpub.com	CANADA	
www.jbpub.com		

Jones and Bartlett's books and products are available through most bookstores and online booksellers. To contact Jones and Bartlett Publishers directly, call 800-832-0034, fax 978-443-8000, or visit our website, www.jbpub.com.

Substantial discounts on bulk quantities of Jones and Bartlett's publications are available to corporations, professional associations, and other qualified organizations. For details and specific discount information, contact the special sales department at Jones and Bartlett via the above contact information, or send an email to specialsales@jbpub.com.

Production Credits
Chief Executive Officer: Clayton Jones
Chief Operating Officer: Don W. Jones, Jr.
President, Higher Education and Professional Publishing: Robert W. Holland, Jr.
V.P., Sales and Marketing: William J. Kane
V.P., Design and Production: Anne Spencer
V.P., Manufacturing and Inventory Control: Therese Connell
Executive Publisher: Christopher Davis
Special Projects Editor: Elizabeth Platt
Associate Editor: Kathy Richardson
Associate Marketing Manager: Laura Kavigian
Cover Design: Kate Ternullo
Cover Image: ©Photos.com
Printing and Binding: Malloy Inc.
Cover Printing: Malloy Inc.

Library of Congress Cataloging-in-Publication Data

Sheremata, William A.
　100 questions & answers about multiple sclerosis / William A. Sheremata.
　　p. cm.
　Includes index.
　ISBN 0-7637-4763-7 (pbk.)
　1. Multiple sclerosis. I. Title: One hundred questions and answers about multiple sclerosis. II. Title.
　RC377.S55 2006
　616.8'34--dc22

　　　　　　　　　　　　　　2005036042

6048
Printed in the United States of America
09 08 07 06 05　　10 9 8 7 6 5 4 3 2 1

Contents

Part 1. The Basics   *3*

Questions 1–15 provide fundamental information about multiple sclerosis, including:

- What is multiple sclerosis?
- What is a lesion?
- What is white matter?

Part 2. Symptoms   *15*

Questions 16–22 describe common symptoms of multiple sclerosis, such as:

- What are the most common symptoms of MS?
- Why am I so fatigued?
- How long do symptoms of MS last?

Part 3. Diagnosis, Identification, and Prognosis   *27*

Questions 23–37 describe diagnosis, identification, and prognosis of different forms of MS, including:

- How is a diagnosis of MS made?
- What kinds of MS exist?
- Do all people with MS become disabled?

Part 4. Causes of Multiple Sclerosis   *47*

Questions 38–56 discuss factors that contribute to development of MS, such as:

- Do viruses cause MS?
- What is the role of the immune system in MS?
- Is MS hereditary?

For most patients, living with multiple sclerosis can be frightening and often devastating. Unfortunately, there are many physicians who are so busy that they lose sight of what the patient is experiencing. Especially in this time of managed care, the average practitioner must increase the volume of patient visits in order to achieve adequate compensation for his long investment of studies, and the patient is left to flounder among often conflicting information without the guidance of a seasoned and caring health provider.

In our information age, people are bombarded with much chatter, often far beyond their ability to put it all together in a meaningful way and all too frequently alarming them to the worst possible outcomes. The field of neuroimmunology, the science behind MS and its treatment, is becoming constantly more complex. Even busy neurologists usually cannot be conversant with the burgeoning knowledge in this field. It thus falls to the academic super-specialist to bridge many branches of science in order to maintain understanding of advances as they occur.

Professor Sheremata has brought us, in this small volume, not only many years of ongoing study but also deep compassion and understanding for the experience of his patients, allowing a first hand view of what an ideal doctor-patient relationship should be. He has presented the concerns of his patients and demonstrates the actual interaction with them, bringing to bear his extensive experience as an MS expert and his knowledge of the latest achievements in this rapidly progressing field. He inspires confidence and reassurance that there is a light at the end of the tunnel and that his charges are not left without hope. He takes up the difficult task of giving clear and easily understandable explanations to the many questions brought to him. Thus, like the model for the caring physician, Maimonides, Dr. Sheremata has provided a fresh approach that will serve as a guide for the bewildered.

Gerard M. Lehrer, MD
December 3, 2005

Multiple sclerosis (MS) is a recent illness in the history of mankind. Although before the latter part of the 19th century several people may have had MS, the first person afflicted with reasonable certainty was Sir Augustus d'Este, a grandson of King George III of England. He was born in 1794, 18 years after the American Declaration of Independence. It was through a detailed diary that Douglas Firth recognized the illness and subsequently published extracts from that diary in 1947 (Cambridge University Press). In the mid 19th century in Paris, Jean-Marie Charcot, the first professor of neurology, recognized the key manifestations of MS and the characteristic pathologic changes in the nervous system. In turn, Charcot attributed the recognition of the illness and tissue changes of MS to Cruveilhier, the renowned professor of anatomy. Sigmund Freud, at that time a student under Charcot, became interested in the emotional aspects of MS.

Regardless of whomever was the first patient affected or who originally described the illness, MS is a uniquely human disease. No comparable natural illness afflicts animals. Experimental models of MS that rely upon diseases in animals, such as experimental allergic encephalomyelitis (EAE), all fall short for many reasons. For the most part, the study of EAE has successfully provided information about immune responses that have been important to human illness, but the specific relevance of EAE to MS has been much more limited.

Important new insights have recently been achieved through the detailed examination of MS brain tissue. Many studies have confirmed Charcot's original ideas of a central role for myelin in MS. Myelin is a fat-laden tissue that surrounds nerve fibers, allowing them to conduct messages from one nerve cell to another at high speeds. Newer studies, using older and more reliable but more expensive techniques, have shown that extensive myelin damage is commonly present in MS but is often not seen in routine brain magnetic resonance imaging (MRI) scans. Other recent studies have refocused interest on the importance of nerve fiber damage and loss in MS in the development of disability. Additional information has come from studies of a newly recognized myelin protein (MOG) and the ability of immune reactions to this protein to produce monkey models of disease more closely resembling the human disease MS. There is hope that these new findings may result in a laboratory test that will help confirm the diagnosis at the onset of the illness. More importantly, these studies are providing new leads as to the cause of MS. Hopefully they will lead to new specific forms of immunotherapy.

The variety of symptoms and neurologic problems in MS can be bewildering for patients and physicians alike. Compounding this complexity is the emotional reaction of patients with MS to their symptoms. The difficulty in arriving at a diagnosis leads to frustration and anxiety for patients. This is also aggravated by fears (many times unrealistic) of imminent disability. The economic implications of the cost of testing and anticipated loss of income engender concern. The presence of anxiety in patients sometimes prompts them to place undue stress on certain symptoms, leading physicians to conclude that the problem is related to anxiety alone. In my experience, approximately two of three women ultimately found to have MS were initially diagnosed as being anxious, depressed, or "hysterical."

Many drugs, especially antidepressant and sedative drugs, may affect both symptoms of MS and neurologic functions. Over-the-counter drugs such as dolomite (lithium carbonate), for example, impact both emotional control and immune function. Unfounded claims for a host of substances in health food stores and mail-order sources are legion. The promised benefits may be lacking, but toxicities of many products are real.

Answers to the question "what is MS?" will differ greatly depending on who is asking the question and who is answering. A physician has a perspective of MS that will depend on his or her education and clinical experience. The physician's view may include views of scientists who study the changes in normal anatomy and function of the human nervous system. Moreover, practicing physicians may see the question differently when they are trained in general neurology. When trained in the subspecialty of MS, their insight may be quite different. The perspective of the physician trained in psychology or psychiatry may also differ markedly, but in the end, all these views are meaningful to the patient.

Patients often define the question "what is MS?" from their own particular concerns, which are in a different realm from those of health care professionals. These patients' concerns are often focused on specific issues, such as their perception that these symptoms represent a threat to their own physical independence. Their immediate worry is about outcomes of specific symptoms or limitations that they may already have. The perspectives of the patient and physician may intersect later. Often, when the informed patient has his or her original issues addressed, then he or she will have a better understanding of the scientific underpinnings of the illness and outcomes of research as they relate to treatment options.

Hopefully, the response to the question "What is MS?" in this book will be meaningful to readers. This question has been addressed from a number of different overlapping perspectives asked by a variety of patients with different educational backgrounds and disease manifestations. Dozens of patients have been asked what their most important question about MS was and what they thought the answer should address. An effort was made to address the specific question they were asking. Many patients were college graduates, whereas others had not graduated from high school. Nevertheless, their questions and concerns were similar. The question *What is Multiple Sclerosis?* was asked by almost two thirds of the patients who submitted their questions for this book.

William A. Sheremata, MD, FRCPC, FACP

This book, *100 Questions & Answers About Multiple Sclerosis*, is dedicated to the many patients who submitted their questions that I have attempted to answer, as well as the many others whom I have served for more than three decades. The questions used in the book were actual questions that patients and their families asked. Many patients asked the same questions, sometimes using different words and from different perspectives. The answers are organized pretty much in the same fashion as the other books in the *100 Questions & Answers* series.

The influence of two people on my career must be acknowledged. The first is Norman Geschwind, MD, who was the Putnam Professor of Neurology at Harvard. This "Renaissance man" stimulated me to pursue laboratory research in neuroimmunology as well as clinical training in neurology at the Boston VAH and Boston City Hospitals. The second is James Bertrand Cosgrove, MD, at the Montreal Neurological Institute, who, despite my protests, patiently cultivated my clinical skills and broadened my knowledge of multiple sclerosis.

I am indebted to Karen Miller for her enthusiastic response to my invitation to review, reflect, and comment on the content of this book. Over the last eight years I have gotten to know and respect Karen and her husband David through interactions in our MS Center. Karen is an exceptionally intelligent, altruistic, and caring woman. With the help of her family she has accepted her diagnosis and adjusted her life in response to MS, interrupting her flourishing and gifted legal career to focus on MS. She participated in a Phase II study of Tysabri and became an enthusiastic proponent for the treatment based on her personal experience. Throughout the last eight years she has been fortunate to have a supportive family.

The indulgence, patience, and assistance of my family in completing this book is acknowledged and is deeply appreciated.

William A. Sheremata, MD, FRCPC, FACP

PART ONE

The Basics

What is multiple sclerosis?

Where does MS occur in the nervous system?

What is a lesion?

More...

1. What is multiple sclerosis?

Multiple sclerosis
a neurologic disease that is characterized by focal demyelination in the central nervous system, lymphocytic infiltration in the brain, with a variably progressive course.

Central nervous system (CNS)
the term CNS refers to the brain and spinal cord.

In the classic sense, **multiple sclerosis** (MS) is a *disease* of the **central nervous system** (the brain and spinal cord) that most commonly affects young adults. *Sclerosis* means hardening; MS means that there are multiple areas of hardened tissue in the brain and spinal cord. The word *disease* means a loss of a feeling of ease (i.e., *dis-ease*), or otherwise stated, a loss of a sense of well-being. This is a meaningful definition for MS patients faced with a bewildering variety of other specific symptoms. Often, patients afflicted with MS have difficulty describing just how they feel. Although the MS patient appreciates and understands this concept, many healthy persons, including physicians, unfortunately, often do not.

Neurologist
a physician specializing in the diagnosis and care of neurological disease.

The **neurologist** recognizes MS as a disease with many different symptoms that come and go, thus affecting different parts of the nervous system. To be considered as a manifestation of MS (an attack), a symptom should last at least 1 day (24 hours). Any of the presenting problems of MS may appear singly or in combination. Some of the symptoms can be evidence of other illnesses unrelated to MS.

The question "what is MS?" is like the proverbial blind men and the elephant: the description depends on the individual experience. The following questions have been arranged to help you build a working knowledge of what this illness is.

Karen's comment:

My MS is my MS. Each person who has MS has different symptoms, different manifestations of the same symptom, and different ways of dealing with (or not!) the illness. I hope that my remarks are of help to someone somehow, but I do not claim to know what is best for anyone else with MS. Indeed, many times I am not certain even for myself.

Unlike what MS is, I do have a sense of what MS is not. For me, MS is not a blessing. MS is not a curse. MS is not my fault. MS is not something that anyone could have prevented, and MS is not an excuse. Perhaps, most importantly, MS is not the end of my ability to live and to love.

2. Where does MS occur in the nervous system?

All of the symptoms and abnormalities that the neurologists found on the neurologic examination and that are thought to be evidence of MS are the result of **lesions** of the brain and the spinal cord. The loss of well-being is probably the consequence of the **immune system** becoming activated.

3. What is a lesion?

Physicians often use the term lesion to indicate focal tissue damage in some part of the body. MS symptoms that neurologists are "tuned into" are the consequence of **inflammation** in the nervous system. Inflammation occurs in spots that are scattered in the brain and spinal cord that are called **plaques**. If these are large enough, they usually show up in brain or spinal cord **magnetic resonance imaging** (**MRI**) scans.

Lesion
localized area of tissue damage.

Immune system
the host defense against infection comprised of the white blood cells circulating in the blood and other tissues (including the bone marrow), lymph nodes, and the thymus.

Inflammation
the accumulation of fluid, plasma proteins, and white blood cells initiated by physical injury, infection, or local immune response.

Plaque
the plate-like hardened areas of myelin damage and scarring in MS located in the brain and spinal cord.

Magnetic resonance imaging (MRI)
imaging of the brain obtained by the use of magnetic fields and radio frequency together with computerized tomography

4. What is a plaque?

These spots of inflammation and scarring responsible for the hardening are often called plaques and are found in the **white matter** of the brain and spinal cord. They are called plaques because they looked like little plates to Charcot, the French doctor who first found them more than a century ago. Plaque is the French word for plate. They may also occur in the **optic nerve**, which is actually part of the brain and not really a "nerve."

5. What is white matter?

The outermost layer of the brain is the **cortex** or **gray matter**, which is made up of brain cells (**neurons**). The cortex completely covers the white matter, which is the greatest part of the brain and serves to connect different neurons. The neurons in the cortex send nerve fibers (**axons**) to and receive axons from other parts of the brain and spinal cord.

White matter is largely made of myelin and gets its name because it has a lot of fat in it and looks whitish. Although MRI pictures allow us to identify areas of damage in the white matter of the brain or spinal cord, they actually show us areas of increased water in the brain. MRI scans in this way identify areas of inflammation or scarring from previous damage. These areas of damage that are seen may be plaques that MS caused or may be the result of some other disease process. It has recently been clearly shown that damage to myelin that is not caused by inflammation will not show up in an ordinary MRI brain scan (Figures 1 and 2).

Axons are damaged by the inflammatory process, and some are lost permanetly. This loss of axons is thought to be important in the development of disability and disease progression.

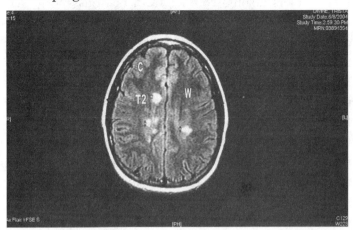

Figure 1. MRI of the brain. A transverse section shows "T2" bright spots in the white matter (labeled "W") of the brain. Note the cortex ("C"), the slightly lighter gray area in the image, which is the layer over the white matter. The bright T2 areas are often referred to by physicians as "hyper-intense areas T2 signal" and at other times are simply called plaques.

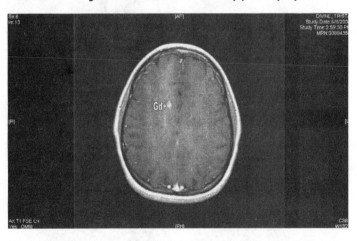

Figure 2. MRI of the same brain shown in Figure 1. A transverse section shows a smaller bright area labeled "Gd+" in a different type of MRI. This is a "T1 weighted" image with an "enhancing" lesion that appeared after gadolinium was injected intravenously. The areas that were bright in Figure 1 are not bright in this image. The enhancing lesion is evidence of active inflammation present at the time of the MRI scan. Note that the enhancing lesion is a small portion of one of the T2 lesions shown in Figure 1. This means that only part of the bright area in Figure 1 is "active" and is added onto a pre-existing plaque.

6. What is myelin?

Nerve fibers (axons) coming from neurons and going to other neurons are surrounded by **myelin**. The axons and the myelin that cover them make up the white matter. Myelin insulates the nerve fibers just like insulation on copper wires. This insulation is important because it speeds up the communication between different areas of the brain. Myelin allows a signal to travel the length of a football field in one second. The plaques of inflammation are areas of damage to myelin and therefore interfere with the function of axons to send messages. Although symptoms of MS will depend on the location of the plaque, many plaques in the brain will not cause any obvious neurologic symptoms (Figure 3).

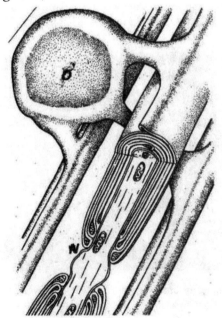

Figure 3. An oligodendrocyte is labeled as "O" in the upper left hand of the drawing. Three of many arm-like extensions of the cell are shown in this drawing. Each of these extensions wrap around separate areas of individual axons, forming myelin sheaths. The myelin sheath is cut away (labeled as N) showing a bulging bit of axon between two myelin sheaths. (After Bunge, 1968).

7. What are "oligos?"

Myelin on the nerve fibers (axons) is arranged like beads on a necklace. The cells that make myelin are called oligodendrocytes. Each of these **oligodendrocytes** sends up to two dozen tentacle-like arms to jelly roll-like nodes of myelin separated by little gaps. Myelin is very important because it helps fibers save 99% of the energy that they would otherwise have to expend. Damage to myelin alone results in messages becoming blocked at the site of damage. Inflammation itself can damage the nerve fiber directly, although there is almost always accompanying myelin damage. Recovery from an attack of MS, at least early recovery, is probably the result of inflammation subsiding. Repair to the axon and myelin may occur within limits.

8. What causes the inflammation in the plaque?

Inflammation in the nervous system is usually caused by **white blood cells** (WBCs), called **lymphocytes** (mostly CD4+ cells); **monocytes** (**macrophages**) from the blood stream usually cause inflammation in the nervous system. Cells and fluids in the blood are normally restricted from entering the nervous system by the blood-brain barrier. This is formed by endothelial cells lining the venules with "tight junctions" uniquely occurring in the brain and spinal cord. A second layer of "foot processes" from astrocytes (star-like cells) buttresses this barrier. In the process of inflammation, these WBCs eat holes through the lining of the smallest blood vessels (venules) and enter the nervous system. Lymphocytes and macrophages are not normally present in the nervous system. However, in some patients, a different type of immune reaction occurs

Oligodendrocyte
glial cells that give rise to the myelin sheath. Each cell forms several myelin sheaths.

White blood cells
leukocytes of the blood. A general term used for all white blood cells including lymphocytes, polymorphonuclear leukocytes, and monocytes.

Lymphocytes
citizens of the immune system.

Macrophages
monocytes from the blood stream that have been "turned on" by interacting with lymphocytes.

Monocytes
part of the human immune system that protects against infections and moves quickly to sites of infection. Monocytes are responsible for phagocytosis, or digestion, of foreign substances in the body.

The Basics

Antibody

proteins made by the immune system to defend against infectious agents. At times, antibody may be directed against our own tissues, resulting in autoimmune disease. Antibody is produced when B-cells are stimulated by antigen.

where antibody is important in damaging myelin. In some, **antibody** may be the sole cause of myelin damage. In another group of patients with a different variation of MS, antibody damage may lead to additional damage that another kind of lymphocyte (CD8+ cells) causes. In ordinary cases of MS, it is not yet clear how important CD8-mediated damage is.

9. What is a macrophage?

Macrophages (meaning "big eaters") are actually monocytes from the blood stream that have been "turned on" by interacting with lymphocytes, which themselves have been turned on by other macrophages that have encountered a foreign protein. These cells have an amazing appetite and ability to damage tissue. For example, in **tuberculosis**, macrophages cause the tissue damage to lungs and other tissues.

Tuberculosis

the disease that results from infection by Mycobacterium tuberculosis. Although most commonly affecting the lungs, any tissue in the body can be involved.

In MS, as seen in Figures 4 and 5, macrophages appear to be the primary cause of myelin damage. Using an electron microscope, you can see actual chunks of myelin inside macrophages in plaques.

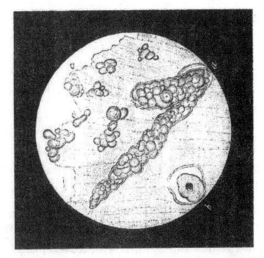

Figure 4. A drawing of a plaque by Charcot using a simple microscope. Charcot described the illustration as "Patch of sclerosis in the fresh state. Lymphatic sheath of a vessel distended by voluminous fatty globules." The fat-laden cells are surrounding a tiny blood vessel in an MS plaque and the cells are filled with myelin. These cells are actually macrophages that have damaged myelin, resulting in "demyelination."

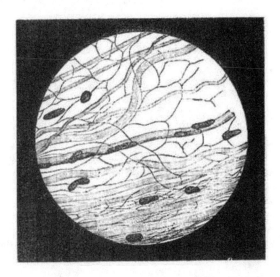

Figure 5. Another drawing by Charcot showing loss of normal myelin around a small blood vessel. This blood vessel is a venule with five or six long, bean-like nuclei oriented more or less vertically in the middle of the drawing. Also seen are spaghetti-like axons without myelin, which appear smaller than the other axons with their myelin intact. This observation led to multiple sclerosis being termed a "demyelinating disease."

10. How do the white blood cells get into the brain and spinal cord?

When lymphocytes become turned on by an immune reaction, they, in turn, "turn on" or "activate" blood monocytes. Once activated, monocytes become macrophages and develop incredible appetites. The activated lymphocytes and macrophages have "Velcro-like" molecules on them called **adhesion molecules**. When these cells stick to the inside of the tiniest blood vessels that have corresponding adhesion molecules, they then become able to eat their way through the vessel into the nervous system (Figure 6).

Adhesion molecules
velcro-like proteins on the surface of white blood and other cells that allow them to stick to the lining of veins.

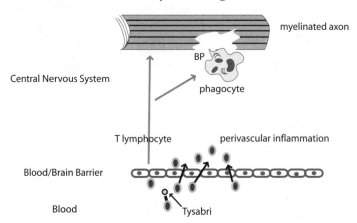

Figure 6. Immunopathogenesis of MS. Mechanisms of demyelination are shown diagrammatically in this illustration. Cells (lymphocytes and macrophages) cross the blood-brain barrier and enter the brain and spinal cord (the central nervous system). These cells then damage myelin. Myelin antibody may also play some role in demyelination. MBP is a major protein component of myelin; Tysabri stops these cells from attaching to the cerebral endothelium and crossing. Note the tight junctions of the endothelium.

11. Can inflammation and plaques be stopped?

Treatment can reduce or even prevent inflammation. The use of **adrenocorticotrophic hormone (ACTH)**, **steroids**, "**ABC**" (Avonex, Betaseron, and Copaxone), and certain other drugs is aimed at stopping or reversing inflammation. These drugs do this in a number of different ways (i.e., they have a number of different actions) that contribute to this end. The use of these drugs is discussed in the section dealing with treatment.

12. At what age do people get MS?

MS has been described as the most common illness causing disability under the age of 45 years. Most people, especially women, have their first symptoms and are diagnosed before the age of 30 years. However, one of five MS patients will have onset of their illness and will be diagnosed after the age of 45 years. This is equally true from the West Coast of Canada to South Florida.

13. Do women get MS more often than men?

Yes, women do get MS more often than men. Approximately 70% of all of the patients diagnosed with MS are women. This is even more so for women under the age of 30 years. Almost four of every five persons with onset of illness under the age of 30 years will be women. In contrast, the onset of MS after the age of 40 years is slightly more common in men.

ACTH

adrenocorticotrophic hormone (now also called cortcotrophin), the hormone made in the brain and stored in the pituitary gland at the base of the brain. It is the only FDA-approved treatment for shortening MS attacks.

Steroids

a large family of chemical substances, including many hormones, chemically defined as containing a tetracyclic cyclopenta alpha phenanthrene skeleton.

"ABC"

a commonly used, unofficial reference to Avonex-Betaseron-Copaxone as approved drugs for MS treatment.

The Basics

Demyelinating disease

diseases caused by demyelination. Disease primarily associated with damage to myelin, e.g., acute disseminated encephalomyelitis and MS.

Estrogen

the steroid produced by the ovary that is responsible for the secondary sexual characteristics of adult females.

The reason for MS occurring more frequently in women than in men is unknown. Female experimental animals develop **demyelinating disease** more predictably and of greater severity than males. This and the fact that women have decreased disease activity during pregnancy suggest that sex hormones influence disease activity. The finding that a hormone, which is a "placental **estrogen**," has a favorable effect in women with MS supports this theory. The administration of this oral estrogen prevented new active brain lesions in a recent MRI study.

14. Does MS affect people of different races differently?

Most of the people with MS are of European descent. MS is less common in African Americans (about half as common) and appears to be even less common among Asians living in the United States. These observations are in agreement with the finding that MS is rare in Africa and in Asia. However, in Australia, a country that is populated predominantly by people of European descent, MS is less common than in the United States, Canada, and Europe. Also, a so-called "North–South gradient" (explained in Question 15) is apparently seen in Australia.

15. How does latitude affect MS?

Observations that MS is more common in the Northern latitudes of Europe and North America were originally interpreted as showing a latitude effect, the so-called North–South gradient. Recent evidence suggests that this may be an artifact that caused immigration patterns. Emigrating Northern (European) peoples originally settled in northern latitudes in America that more closely resembled their homelands. It has been found that veterans with Scandinavian surnames living in the northern United States have the same risk of MS as those who live in the South. In the past, few neurologists lived in the southern United States. This was and still is true in areas of Australia. Because a diagnosis is not accepted unless made by a neurologist, it is obviously made less commonly in underserved areas such as northern Australia and, at least in the past, the southern United States.

The Basics

PART TWO

Symptoms

What are the symptoms of MS? Which symptoms
are most common?

Why am I so fatigued?

How long do the symptoms of MS last?

More...

16. What are the symptoms of MS? Which symptoms are most common?

Symptoms of MS vary from common problems such as unexplained difficulty in walking (occurring in about half of patients at the very beginning) to those that are relatively less common, such as blurred vision, to truly uncommon symptoms such as repeated sudden and brief spasms in one or more limbs (paroxysmal **dystonia**).

Despite the many different medical problems that can cause walking difficulty, the experienced neurologist assumes that a young person using a cane most likely has MS. Also, when someone is diagnosed with **optic neuritis** (or **retrobulbar neuritis**), we know that the vast majority of patients will be diagnosed with MS within 15 years. Approximately half of those affected by optic neuritis will have another episode of neurologic difficulty within a year. If they see an experienced neurologist, they will then be diagnosed with "clinically definite MS."

There are so many different symptoms of MS that it is almost meaningless to list them. Nevertheless, almost all of these difficulties can occur in other neurologic diseases. It is the relapsing-remitting character of symptoms that is the best evidence that any particular neurologic manifestation is caused by MS. The appearance of neurologic problems such as difficulty in walking (i.e., the "attack") followed by improvement (i.e., the "remission") is what characterizes MS in the typical patient.

Dystonia

abnormal muscle tone usually resulting in an abnormal position (posture) relative to the rest of the body.

Optic neuritis (retrobulbar neuritis)

an inflammation of the optic nerve with pain and variable loss of vision. Most patients will eventually be diagnosed as having MS.

A neurologist is required to make a diagnosis of MS, but the diagnosis may be difficult in some patients. In the past, the diagnosis of MS was usually delayed for many years. Two decades ago, the typical delay in diagnosis in the United States was 7 years or more, and in the United Kingdom, it was up to 11 years. This should not happen in this day and age.

Difficulty walking is the most commonly recognized difficulty in MS when first seen by a physician and occurs in about half of the patients at the outset of their illness. This is often due to mild weakness or stiffness of one leg, although sometimes both legs are affected. It is rather common to have the difficulty appear during more prolonged physical activity and particularly with heat exposure. Both raise body temperature and bring out symptoms in MS. Balance problems may also present as gait difficulty.

Actually, numbness and tingling in one or both hands or feet is probably the most common symptom. However, the patient or the physician may not seriously consider them as evidence of illness without other accompanying symptoms. It is general knowledge that otherwise normal people may occasionally have these transient symptoms. A neurologist should investigate if numbness or tingling with or without any other symptom lasts a full day or longer. Recurrent numbness over a period of time is of equal importance.

Difficulties with coordination or the appearance of **tremor** should always be considered as evidence of nervous system disease and should be investigated. In

Tremor
an oscillating rhythmic movement usually involving an extremity. Head movement may accompany tremor but is termed titubation.

Nystagmus

fine rhythmic oscillating movements of the eyeball.

Charcot's triad

the collection of symptoms includes nystagmus, dysarthria, and tremor (shakey eyes, slurred speech, and shaking of the hands and body) that was described as being characteristic of MS. Although occurring in MS, it is rare.

Glaucoma

the disease of the eye characterized by increased intraocular pressure causing damage to the retina and impaired vision.

Trigeminal neuralgia

intense, brief, facial pain typically occurring on one side. It is uncommon before 65 years of age, except in MS. Its occurrence in young adults is usually a sign of MS.

the past, some neurologists would not make a diagnosis without the presence of tremor, shaky eyes (**nystagmus**), and difficulty in speaking, the so-called "**Charcot's triad.**" However, only a minority of patients will ever develop these symptoms; when present, it signals the presence of particularly severe disease.

Although visual problems are less common at onset of illness, they become relatively common over the lifetime of patients with untreated MS. A physician should always evaluate visual symptoms, especially double vision or blurring of vision accompanied by pain in one or both eyes. MS-caused blindness is uncommon. **Glaucoma** is a more common cause of blindness.

Karen's comment:

When I thought I had a problem with a tooth, it turned out to be MS. It took the dentist, an x-ray, and my sister's research about **trigeminal neuralgia** *to convince me that the overwhelming pain in my face was MS. When I had a tightness in my chest, it turned out to be MS. It took a heart specialist, my wearing a heart monitor, and several heart exams to reassure my neurologist and my husband that the extra heartbeats were MS. When I lost my vision, it turned out to be MS. When I forgot what year it was, it turned out to be MS . . . and so on.*

If I have a new medical problem, it is appropriate to rule out non-MS causes. Sometimes a sore tooth, extra heartbeats, blurry vision, memory lapses, skin growths, and a raspy throat are what they would be for someone without MS. However, more often than not, the new (and some-

times weird) symptom can be traced to a brain, nerve, or muscle cell that fires, misfires, or stops firing because of MS. With approximately 10 billion brain cells, 45 miles of nerves, and 650 muscles, if something is wrong with me, the odds are that it is MS.

17. Why am I so fatigued?

Fatigue (a lack of energy) is a common and important manifestation of MS and is even more common than numbness and tingling. Although not specific to MS, it occurs in the vast majority of patients. Many report that it is their major problem. Increased fatigue accompanies most attacks of MS and is an important factor aggravating other manifestations of MS. In actuality, when many patients complain of "fatigue," they often are referring to **fatigability**. A typical example of this occurs when a patient begins walking without difficulty, but after a hundred yards or so must either hold onto another person or object or must stop. A large number of patients run out of energy by midday and must stop and rest. An unexplained severe lack of energy often precedes other symptoms with the onset of an attack of MS.

Most physicians, including neurologists, find it difficult or impossible to assess fatigue. Therefore, scoring systems for quantifying this complaint have been developed to help evaluate its response to treatment. Some physicians use these "fatigue scales," but others reject them as being "too subjective." Fatigue responds to certain drugs, but in contrast, fatigability often requires limitation and pacing of physical activity. It is important to distinguish these terms because "fatigue," as defined by social security, is actually fatigability and

Fatigue

a lack of energy and motivation. It is a common symptom in MS and other autoimmune disorders.

Fatigability

the loss of muscle strength following repeated use or testing of one or more muscles.

21

is a criterion for the evaluation of disability. The proper use of the **extended disability scoring system (EDSS)** by a neurologist experienced in its use is a valid way of evaluating "fatigue" (fatigability).

Extended Disability Scoring System (EDSS)

a grading scale for recording levels of neurological disability. It is used universally for recording disability.

18. How long do the symptoms of MS last?

To be considered a symptom of MS, the symptom should last at least 24 hours. However, certain rare symptoms such as recurrent brief spasms in one or more limbs can be recognized as part of MS (paroxysmal dystonia). Although they are of short duration, typically seconds to minutes, they are identified because they recur in a stereotyped fashion. Other symptoms, such as the loss of muscle tone, difficulty with articulation during speaking, pain, and so on, may be due to MS.

Symptoms in MS typically develop over a period of several days but rarely evolve over more than 2 or 3 weeks. They typically dissipate over a much longer period of time than they appeared, often over a period of weeks and sometimes months. Rest certainly shortens the duration of symptoms. Before the advent of ACTH treatment for MS a half a century ago, rest was the only effective treatment, as it was in tuberculosis since the days of Hippocrates in ancient Greece.

Karen's comment:

Some of my symptoms have lasted a few days, and some have lasted for 6 months. The symptom that I have had last the longest is vertigo. When I moved certain ways or people and objects moved, it triggered severe dizziness, the room spinning, me feeling like I was spinning, and accompanying nausea. The banners on a TV screen, cars on the road, ceiling fans, and my husband moving his fork at dinner are examples of what I had to avoid seeing. Thus, I stayed indoors. I listened to recorded books. I ate meals next to rather than across from my husband-all compensatory processes. As time went on, the accidental triggers occurred less, but the points at which I felt I could not live with the vertigo occurred more.

The vertigo started suddenly and ended quickly. Eight months later, I felt dizzy again. I sobbed, thinking that I was going to have another long bout, but it turned out to be just the flu. When I did have the next episode of vertigo, I thought it would never end. However, like many symptoms, with time, it did.

19. Is my stuttering due to my MS?

Stuttering is not part of MS. However, intermittent difficulty with speech was recognized as a rare manifestation of MS 40 years ago (paroxysmal **dysarthria**). This difficulty with articulation is often associated with difficulty in finding the "right" word. It is rarely recognized as a manifestation of MS, and many doctors incorrectly regard it as an emotional problem. Misdiagnosis is unfortunate because this disorder is amenable to treatment. There are a number of other brief (typically seconds to minutes) recurrent stereotyped paroxysmal (short duration) manifestations that rarely accompany MS. Sometimes they are mistaken as **seizures** but respond to anticonvulsant (antiseizure) treatment as if they were seizures. However, they do not require life-long drug therapy but rather long-term (3 to 6 months) treatment. These manifestations of MS usually respond to lower doses of drugs, doses that

Dysarthria
slurred speech.

Seizure
an epileptic event consisting of loss of consciousness usually associated with tonic and/or clonic movements.

would not control seizures. Tegretol (carbamazepine) is effective in small doses. The drug is well tolerated, is relatively inexpensive, and is my drug of choice. It is beyond the scope of this book to discuss these issues further.

20. How severe are attacks of MS?

The manifestations of MS are often mild and transient but less commonly may be severe. Shortly after the discovery of MS as a disease in Paris, Uhthoff, a Viennese physician, found that increases in body temperature could temporarily result in blurred vision in a young man who had recovered from an attack of optic neuritis. This ("Uhthoff") phenomenon can also result in other symptoms occurring transiently (or as long as body temperature is increased). It is important to know that these *increases in symptoms brought out by elevating body temperature are* **not** *attacks of MS.* However, if the same symptoms occur in the absence of a fever or elevated body temperature, they may be mild attacks of MS.

Attacks of MS can sometimes be severe and require a prolonged period of recovery lasting as long as a year or so, but this is unusual. ACTH and high-dose intravenous (IV) steroids shorten the period of recovery; however, many attacks are mild, and treatment is not needed. Fortunately, effective treatments (high doses of **interferon**-beta, Betaseron, or Rebif) for MS reduce the risk of these severe attacks more than milder attacks. In the studies that led to Food and Drug Administration (FDA) approval, interferon-beta reduced the frequency of severe attacks by almost 50% as compared with a 30% overall reduction. This is

Interferons

cytokines; proteins made by lymphocytes that can induce cells to resist viral replication.

24

more meaningful when you realize that severe attacks are associated with an inability to function and are usually treated in hospital.

Karen's comment:

Closely correlated with the maxim "if it is a symptom, it is probably MS" is "if it is an MS symptom, it is not necessarily a new attack." MS is finely balanced and disrupted by medications and changes in my body. Things that seem straightforward or completely unrelated to MS may affect MS and require input from the neurologist. I have learned to ask Dr. Sheremata if he approves of something I want to do. The answer is sometimes yes, sometimes no, sometimes if you must, and sometimes the glasses are lowered and a look of disbelief crosses his face!

21. Can I go blind with MS?

Although visual loss accompanying attacks of MS, diagnosed as optic neuritis or retrobulbar neuritis, may occasionally be severe, blindness is unusual. There may be a small blind spot left after an attack, and occasionally, this may be large enough to interfere with vision. Glaucoma, which is another type of eye disease, unrelated to MS, is more common as a cause of blindness in MS patients.

Karen's comment:

*My vision problems range from a bit of blurriness to a complete lack of sight. I inherited extreme **myopia**; I wear contact lenses and glasses even in the shower. Before MS, changes in my vision required new prescriptions and picking out the least offensive frames. MS vision symptoms and*

Myopia

nearsightedness; inability to see distant objects without corrective lenses.

optic neuritis were entirely new and different experiences for me.

The first time I lost my vision I panicked, certain that it would not return. The second time I panicked less. The third time my family worried less, and the fourth time, I nonchalantly said to myself, "Oh it's just MS, and I've done this before," but I was not entirely reassured. Each time I was very relieved and a bit surprised when my vision returned.

22. What causes walking difficulty in MS?

Difficulty with walking in MS can result from plaques in different places in the brain stem and spinal cord. The location of the plaques determines, in large part, whether that difficulty is due to the particular problems of weakness, loss of sensation, or incoordination of the legs. In certain places in the brain and spinal cord, plaques can produce weakness; those in the back part of the spinal cord cause certain kinds of sensation loss (position sense); others in the **cerebellum** and its connections lead to incoordination in the legs. Any or all of these disturbances can contribute to gait difficulty.

Cerebellum

the part of the brain that controls movement, resulting in coordinated movement. It is located behind the brainstem and under the cerebral hemispheres and resembles a pair of tennis balls stuck to the brain stem.

The most common problem that causes difficulty in walking is "weakness." When a patient complains of "weakness," he or she is often describing one of several different problems. Muscle weakness in nervous system disease is often the result of messages not getting to the muscles from the brain and spinal cord. A signal or message may begin in the brain (the precentral or motor area of the brain), but it has to travel to neurons located in the spinal cord, perhaps up to 3 feet away. The signal travels down a small part of the spinal cord called the **pyramidal tract**.

One or more MS plaques along the way may prevent part, or all, of that message from getting to the neuron, resulting in "weakness" and difficulty standing and walking. The larger the plaque, the more likely it is to interfere with many messages to many neurons and produce more weakness of the muscle these neurons supply.

Sometimes patients complain of weakness, but the examining neurologist may not detect any weakness. What is going on? If he or she watches the person walk, the patient may be seen dragging one leg; if the patient walks up and down the hallway without stopping, this same patient may not be able to walk 100 yards. Repeated examination may reveal a lot of weakness in certain leg muscles.

If different nerve fibers are affected, such as those sensory fibers that send messages to the brain telling it where the legs are, then the person will not be able to control the legs. Movement might occur, but it may be clumsy and poorly controlled and, therefore, not be useful. This is a major problem! The patient's legs may or may not feel "numb."

Another problem that contributes to walking difficulty, especially early in the illness, is a lack of coordination because of a plaque in the cerebellum (that part of the brain just above the spinal cord inside the skull). (The cerebellum looks like a couple of tennis balls stuck together on top of something that looks like a fatter spinal cord.) A plaque in the spinal cord can also

Pyramidal tract
the nerve fiber tract in the brainstem and spinal cord comprised of the nerve fibers arising from the motor cortex.

Symptoms

cut off fibers connecting the cerebellum to neurons in the spinal cord, resulting in gait problems. The patient does not have to have a tremor to have difficulty because of a plaque in the cerebellum or its connections.

In summary, MS plaques can affect several different parts of the brain and spinal cord and cause difficulty in walking.

PART THREE

Diagnosis, Identification, and Prognosis

How is a diagnosis of MS made?

What kinds of MS exist?

Do all people with MS become disabled?

More...

23. How is a diagnosis of MS made?

A diagnosis of MS is not generally accepted unless a neurologist confirms the diagnosis. In actuality, many general physicians are aware of the illness and recognize the characteristic problems that patients have with MS. Some have a heightened awareness of the disease, whereas others are more proficient in carrying out a neurologic exam. However, other than neurologists with subspecialty training in MS, few have the training and experience to carry out a quantitative neurologic examination. Regardless of who the examining physician is, certain diagnostic criteria for MS must be met. The first formal criteria for the diagnosis of MS were outlined in what is commonly called the "Schumacher criteria."

Dr. George Schumacher was the head of a National Institutes of Health committee that was charged with the responsibility of coming up with simple standardized minimal criteria that were to be used in making a diagnosis of MS in patients entering clinical trials in MS. The criteria reiterated the need to establish that the lesions (plaques) were "disseminated in both time and space." In other words, to make a diagnosis of MS, there must be evidence of at least two separate affected areas in the brain and spinal cord, and the lesions must have occurred at least at two different times separated by at least 1 month. Bearing in mind that this preceded diagnostic imaging, this was a challenge.

A little more than 20 years ago the (National Institutes of Health) Poser committee was brought together under the chairmanship of Dr. Charles Poser. This committee recognized that laboratory support for the diagnosis of MS from diagnostic imaging and improvements in **spinal fluid** examination was a major advance. The terms *clinically definite, clinically probable,* and *laboratory-supported* diagnoses come into use in academic circles but were rarely used elsewhere. Nevertheless, the committee recommendations (the *Poser criteria)* focused interest on using MRI as well as spinal fluid **immunoglobulin** abnormalities in the diagnosis of MS. Spinal fluid analysis, however, has suffered from the lack of standardization of diagnostic testing. The FDA is in the process of addressing this issue and has now outlined certain methods that must be used for detection of **oligoclonal bands**. These are bands that appear in the gamma globulin region of spinal fluid during electrophoresis testing in the laboratory. If present, they provide strong support for the diagnosis of MS. This action is required because proper testing is more expensive and the mandate for this testing is needed to ensure appropriate insurance coverage.

Spinal fluid
fluid produced by the choroids plexus within the brain. It is located in the ventricles and surrounds the brain and spinal cord.

Immunoglobulin
another word for antibody.

Oligoclonal band
bands of antibody that are present in electrophoresis of CSF.

Karen's comment:

On December 12, 1996, I began the day as a mostly healthy professor of legal ethics with a nagging case of an "inner ear virus."

I ended the day as an MS patient. In between the start and end of the day, I drove to the university to pick up my students' exams for grading and then to the doctor for him to examine my ears and give me my annual pap test.

During that fall term, I was flying each week between New Jersey where my husband was studying at the Princeton Theological Seminary and Florida where my middle

Virus
pathogens composed of a nucleic acid genome enclosed in a protein coat. Viruses can replicate only in a living cell.

sister, niece, father, and stepmother live. I taught Legal Ethics at New York University School of Law in the north and University of Miami School of Law in the south. For 3 months I had extreme vertigo that was seemingly caused by "an inner ear virus." I reassured myself that when I stopped this crazy schedule, I would heal.

By December I was taking large amounts of Antivert, Dramamine, and ginger ale to get through a 3-hour class. If I moved too fast or a student waved a hand or turned a page of a book without warning, I would fight the nausea that comes from vertigo. I memorized my lectures so that I did not have to look down at my notes. I would sometimes have to vomit during the breaks in class, wash my face, and then continue to teach. On the day I picked up the students' exams to grade, I went to see my general doctor. He immediately said that I did not have a virus and refused to let me drive myself to the emergency appointment he made with a neurologist.

My father took me to the neurologist, who said I had either a large brain tumor or MS and scheduled an MRI for that day as well as a spinal tap for the next day. The MRI center was having a holiday party, and while we waited for the results to take back to the neurologist, the office administrator offered us Santa party hats and snacks to keep us distracted. My husband who was in New Jersey, kept saying, "I thought you were having a pap test and had a problem with your ears. What are you doing at the neurologist?" We were all a bit in shock as the surreal nature of the day continued. With MRI results and party favors in hand, we went back to the neurologist who had waited after hours for our return. He looked at the MRI and said, "You have MS."

The doctor asked whether I had ever had any prior events of weakness or numbness. By the time we went through his questions and my answers, a pattern of unexplained, often ignored, yet classic MS symptoms was evident. Previously, when a medical problem would get too bothersome, I would finally make an appointment with a doctor. Inevitably, the symptom went away; I was too busy to keep the appointment before it went away or an explanation emerged, and thus, I canceled the appointment. I was a typical over-achiever: working, making Christmas decorations by hand, entertaining my husband's corporate clients, starting a soup kitchen at our church, and keeping in touch with family each day. Fatigue was apparently due to hard work at law school and around-the-clock hours as a hostile takeover lawyer in the 1980s. Weakness in my right hand was explained as a side effect from writing a law review article and having a lumpectomy. Changes in my vision were thought to be due to long hours and the water in London causing an occasional film on my contact lenses. The inability to walk on my right foot was apparently from falling off a curb, causing a sprain that lasted 6 months. Other injuries seemingly resulted from general clumsiness, a lack of good depth perception, and so on.

Looking back, I am not sure whether it would have mattered if I had been diagnosed earlier. Over the 20 years before my diagnosis (when I had what I now know were MS symptoms), I had completed college in 3 years, married, graduated from law school, practiced and taught law, lived overseas for 10 years, and planned a family; I had lived a "normal" life. In 1996, after 3 months of severe symptoms and with an MRI showing areas of my brain scarred from prior attacks, MS could no longer be ignored and now loomed large.

24. What is a "clinically isolated syndrome or CIS?"

Transverse myelitis

signs of spinal cord damage appearing acutely or subacutely with signs of inflammation. When accompanied by certain MRI abnormalities, it may qualify for a diagnosis of CIS/MS.

Clinically isolated syndrome (CIS)

optic neuritis, acute vertigo or other isolated brainstem symptoms, or transverse myelitis may be referred to as CIS and may qualify for a diagnosis of MS when certain MRI abnormalities are present.

Acute disseminated encephalomyelitis

an acute spontaneous, postinfectious, or postvaccinial central nervous system disease. It can be very serious but more often is a relatively mild illness.

Neurologists have long recognized optic neuritis (or retrobulbar neuritis) to be a forerunner of MS in the majority of cases. Recognizing this and the fact that other problems such as **transverse myelitis** and acute symptoms of brainstem origin also usually end up diagnosed as MS, the McDonald committee has modified the Poser criteria to establish the *"McDonald criteria."*

These criteria embrace the rational use of laboratory investigation in making the diagnosis of MS and but have abandoned the terms clinically probable and laboratory supported. The committee has simply and clearly outlined MRI criteria that can be used together with a history of a single clinical attack (called **clinically isolated syndrome [CIS])** to make a diagnosis of MS with a high degree of certainty. Approximately one in five or six persons diagnosed with MS based on MRI criteria will not have MS, however. In all probability, most of this small group will have had an attack of **acute disseminated encephalomyelitis** (a one-time "MS" attack). Recent evidence indicates that this kind of attack seems to be related to a different kind of immune reaction. We anticipate that new tests may help to distinguish this group at the onset of illness.

The decision of the committee to include MRI criteria for a CIS and to equate CIS with a diagnosis of MS was, in part, driven by the evidence from two separate studies. These are the CHAMPS study of Avonex and the ETOMS study of Rebif. These studies showed superior results when interferon-beta-1a treatment was started after the very first clinical attack of MS. The

Diagnosis, Identification, and Prognosis

very low dose of Rebif in the ETOMS study yielded inferior results as compared with the CHAMPS study. The FDA has accepted initiation of treatment based on the McDonald criteria, including the "CIS" category.

25. What are the actual new "McDonald diagnostic criteria" that neurologists use to make a diagnosis of MS?

The McDonald committee outlined the criteria in an article titled Recommended Diagnostic Criteria, which is in the *Annals of Neurology*. These criteria have been adopted in the United States and internationally. The summary prepared by the National Multiple Sclerosis Society is presented in Table 1.

TYPES OF MS
26. What kinds of MS exist?

To most physicians dealing with MS and many patients, this illness seems to be a family of closely related disorders. To begin with, a doctor's clinical diagnosis of MS is based on the recognition of symptoms that recur (**relapse**). The relapsing nature of the disease is unique to MS. Recognition of symptoms that are typically associated with MS makes a neurologist's diagnosis easier.

Relapse
appearance of new signs or recurrence of previous signs of MS.

By consensus, MS is usually divided into four different types for the purposes of study: (1) relapsing-remitting MS, (2) secondary progressive MS, (3) primary progressive MS, and (4) relapsing progressive. This does not mean that they have different causes.

Table 1. New MS Diagnostic Criteria

Clinical Attacks	Objective Lesions	Additional Requirements to Make Diagnosis
≥2	≥2	Clinical evidence is enough
≥2	1	Disseminated in space by MRI or +CSF and two more MRI lesions consistent with MS or additional clinical attack in different site
1	2 or more	Disseminated in time by MRI or second clinical attack
1 Mono-symptomatic	1	Disseminated in space by MRI or + CSF and two or more MRI lesions consistent with MS and disseminated in time by MRI or second attack
0 Progressive from start	1	+ CSF and disseminated in space by MRI evidence of three or more T2 brain lesions or two or more cord lesions or four to eight brain and one cord lesions or + VEP and four to eight MS lesions or + VEP and four brain lesions + one cord lesion and disseminated in time by MRI or continued progression for 1 year.

27. If I have relapsing-remitting MS, can I get progressive?

Patients with *relapsing-remitting* illness have attacks of one or more symptoms with varying frequency and with variable degrees of recovery but do not progress between attacks. Relapsing-remitting MS patients have attacks without interval progression, which is the essential feature of this type of MS. If there is progression between attacks, this is *secondary progressive MS*. In contrast, *primary progressive MS* is a type of MS in which patients have no attacks and worsening disease is not followed by subsequent improvement. If primary progressive patients have a subsequent attack with any recovery, they are reclassified as relapsing progressive MS.

It is clear that MS patients can suffer disability but not have secondary progressive, relapsing progressive, or primary progressive MS. No satisfactory terms or descriptors for stepwise progressing MS are in common use.

Rapidly progressive MS or **malignant MS** are terms that are used to describe a small minority of patients who become disabled in a short period of time. These patients typically will have three or more attacks in their first year, often severe, and possess **gene** combinations (HLA-B-7 and DR-2) that occur in a small minority of MS patients. It is particularly important that such patients be provided with expert care in MS clinics because aggressive therapy is the only way to avoid severe permanent disability. Aggressive **immunosuppressive therapy** (**chemotherapy**) with Cytoxan or Novantrone will usually stabilize them. Despite the presence of severe disability when first seen, more than a quarter or more of these patients can experience remarkable improvement. **HIV** screening is important, as rare patients with AIDS can occasionally mimic this type of illness. They do not benefit from the types of treatment that MS patients do.

28. What is chronic progressive MS?

Both secondary progressive and relapsing progressive MS were referred to as *chronic progressive* in the past. The term chronic progressive is no longer used. Primary progressive patients were also sometimes referred to as chronic progressive. Importantly, if an MS

Diagnosis, Identification, and Prognosis

Rapidly progressive MS

a very aggressive form of MS in which the disease advances quickly and relentlessly, leading to rapid disability and death. Also called malignant MS, Marburg's variant of acute MS, or fulminant MS.

Gene

the smallest amount of DNA in chromosomes or mitochondria that codes for a heritable characteristic or feature.

Immunosuppressive therapy

any treatment that results in decreased immune responses.

HIV

human immunodeficiency virus, the AIDS virus.

patient has never had an attack followed by a remission, they are diagnosed as having primary progressive MS. However, if an MS patient begins as a primary progressive but then has an onset of new problems followed by improvement, they then are rediagnosed as "relapsing progressive."

Many neurologists in the past have concluded that there are many more types of MS, but these are not easily characterized or recognized clinically. Therefore, they are no help in determining prognosis or in evaluating the effects of therapy.

Spinal MS

the older term for primary progressive MS, commonly used prior to the modern era of imaging.

Cervical spondylosis

a disease in which the disks between the vertebral bodies in the neck extrude like mortar between bricks. Sometimes the disks will compress the spinal cord, producing "MS-like" symptoms of weakness and loss of sensation in the legs. The disease process can result in pressure on nerve roots as they leave the spinal canal, resulting in weakness and/or pain in the arms and hands.

29. What is spinal MS?

Spinal MS was a term used for primary progressive MS but has not generally been used for the last 30 years or so. It was a good descriptor for this illness because the predominant symptoms were those of slowly progressive weakness and sensory problems, predominantly affecting the legs. In the past, it was especially difficult to distinguish from **cervical spondylosis**. Modern imaging has made this distinction much easier. For the sake of clarity, the term primary progressive MS is preferable.

30. Who gets progressive disease without attacks?

At first, my response was to assume that the person who asked this question was simply asking about the definition of this type of illness. However, he was actually asking about differences in populations and their risk of this type of illness. Here again, ethnic differences become apparent. In France, Charcot first described the spinal form (primary progressive MS) as an "incomplete form" of MS, occurring in about 10% of patients. Subsequently, this form of illness was recognized as occurring in about 30% of Irish patients and later still as occurring in about 30% of the European Jews in Israel. Primary progressive illness also appears to be more common in Spain and in patients of Spanish descent, including Cubans, who live in the United States. Several other disorders must be distinguished from primary progressive MS. The most common of these is cervical spondylosis (compression of the spinal cord because of disc disease). Although people fear spinal cord tumors, only a tiny percentage (about 1%) of patients will be diagnosed as having a spinal cord tumor.

31. How will I know whether I will get progressive disease?

The absence of attacks with new neurologic symptoms, or recurrence of older problems, does not necessarily mean that a person has progressive MS. Patients can be stable for long periods of time. To recognize progression in MS, neurologic difficulties must be progressing. A neurologist can only determine this if the patient has progressed or changed neurologically. The patient must undergo a complete quantitative neurologic examination to determine and then record disability scores for comparison with previous and future examinations. It takes special training to perform such examinations with consistency and to provide usable information. However, the patient with progressive disease can point out to the neurologist what types of problems are progressing.

Reasons why primary progressive patients do not ordinarily have attacks are unknown. Actually, about one third of the patients who originally experience only progressive problems subsequently do experience one or more exacerbations, but when they do, they have relatively few. It is possible that those who never have acute attacks have a different type of disease process that involves antibody-mediated **demyelination** independent of lymphocytes. At the present, this is purely speculative.

Demyelination
the loss of myelin surrounding the axon, or nerve fiber, regardless of the disease process.

In addition to those patients with primary progressive MS, many patients with secondary progressive illness stop having clear-cut attacks and progress in a waxing-and-waning fashion. After a dozen years of illness, progression and attacks may no longer be evident to the patient and physician alike. Evidence of progression by examination may be difficult to detect in many patients. Longer term observation of these patients may reveal continued worsening; that is, neurologic functions that appear to be preserved may actually be partially lost.

PROGNOSIS AND DISABILITY

32. Do all people with MS become disabled?

Some neurologists, many in academic circles, have a perception that MS is predictably associated with disability. Before the advent of new testing procedures, particularly MRI of the brain and spinal cord, many patients were not diagnosed during life. Without proven treatments, there was little incentive to do so in those without disability. The training of many more neurologists in recent years has led to greater availability of neurologic consultation; therefore, a larger proportion of previously undiagnosed patients are now correctly recognized as having MS. Thus, in the past, those who had more evidence of disability than the majority were correctly diagnosed; those who were minimally affected were not. Now that a variety of treatments are available, the importance of early diagnosis and treatment is accepted, and we are seeing a larger number of patients correctly diagnosed as having MS.

In my experience, general physicians previously gave about two thirds of the women who were diagnosed with MS an initial "psychiatric" label. Now, with the advantages of increasing numbers of physicians (neurologists) trained to recognize MS and the general availability of MRI equipment, many more people are recognized as having this disorder. In Europe, where large numbers of patients have been cared for in specialty centers, it is now evident that the majority of these people with MS are not disabled.

33. How long will it be before I will be disabled?

Recently, there has been speculation that disability in MS patients will be predictably present after several years of illness. Some have claimed that there is no difference between various patient groups and that disability eventuates in the majority of patients. Apart from this rhetoric, it is clear that the rate of progression in the early years of illness is in part related to the number of relapses in early illness. The Canadian observation that a single relapse in the first year of illness is a good prognostic sign is one that the majority of neurologists who are experienced in the care of MS share. In the "population studies" in southern Ontario, three attacks in the first year of illness led to wheelchair dependence within 5 years in half of those patients. This is in agreement with the clinical observation that an unusually large number of MS attacks in a short time period predict unusually severe disease.

Genetic studies have shown that patients with aggressive disease are genetically distinguished by the presence of two genes: HLA-B7 and DR-2 (DR-1 1501).

Recent studies of large numbers of patients in Europe, followed and documented for decades, have produced "new" data. These data from Europe indicate that 30% of patients will develop progressive disease rather than a larger estimate from centers here in the United States. It is important to bear in mind that these observations are based primarily on "untreated" MS patients. That is to say, the patients had not benefited from drugs that have been proven to reduce attacks of MS and to reduce the risk of disability.

Large numbers of neurologists interested in MS in the United States, Canada, and Europe have come to the same conclusions regarding the prognosis of MS:

1. Women with MS do better than men!
2. The onset of MS before the age of 30 is associated with a better prognosis.
3. One attack of MS, only, in the first year of illness predicts less disability.

4. Optic neuritis or retrobulbar neuritis as an initial attack has been recognized as being associated with a good prognosis.

5. A low lesion load (numbers of lesions and/or lesion volume) on the MRI has been interpreted as being associated with a better outlook.

34. Why do some people get worse so quickly? Will I?

There are probably many reasons why some people worsen more quickly than others. Stress is implicated in many other diseases, and without question, it plays an important role in MS.

It is clear that some patients are genetically predisposed to rapid progression of illness. Persons who have the DR-2 (DR-1 1501) gene have more severe disease than those who do not. However, Dr. Dupont in Denmark showed 30 years ago that when patients have both the DR-2 gene and HLA-B7, they predictably have rapidly progressive disease and severe disability (malignant MS). For example, in our Florida experience, although only 7% of Cuban patients have the DR-2 gene, when they have both DR-2 and HLB-B7, they too have malignant MS.

There is no simple way of determining beforehand how an individual patient will fare during the course of MS. However, the frequency of attacks (one attack in the first year), good recovery from the attack, a small amount of disease in brain MRI scans, and recovery of a feeling of well-being are good indicators for a better outlook. Treatment has improved the outlook for all MS patients.

35. Is memory affected with MS?

Memory can be affected by MS. Confusion can accompany attacks and can be associated with memory difficulty, but this is not defined as true memory impairment. It is associated with generally impaired **cognition**. Anxiety and/or depression also can rob a person of their ability to maintain attention. When the anxiety or depression abates, memory is again normal. However, memory complaints tend to increase with the duration of illness and disability. The recent Avonex CHAMPS trial documented that early treatment in the course of the illness can prevent cognitive impairment.

Cognition
ability to reason.

Karen's comment:

I used to be smart. When I try to barter with God about my MS, I offer walking in exchange for my memory. When I get sad, angry, depressed, or frustrated with MS, it is usually about my cognitives. When I want my pre–MS self back, it is my intelligence I long for.

In 1996, when I was first diagnosed, I had trouble reading—not surprising given the vertigo, limited vision, and medications. After these symptoms subsided, I still had trouble reading—not problems seeing the words, but rather processing the words. By the time I would finish a page I had no idea what I had read. Cognitive problems were not mentioned or referred to in anything I researched about MS. Dr. Sheremata validated my experience and suggested neuropsychiatric testing to ascertain my cognitive status.

The test results revealed that my long-term memory and even short-term memory were fine, but my short-term working memory was a problem. It was reassuring to know that I was not imagining this, but it was shocking to see the numbers in print—my short-term working memory was in the bottom 16%! What this translates into is difficulty learning new information (phone numbers, names, and places where my things are moved), processing new information (understanding a new or unanticipated item), manipulating information (changing times for an event), making decisions (determining what to have for dinner), and transferring data (addressing an envelope). I can use some other parts of my brain to compensate or almost mask what is occurring, but if I am physically tired or challenged, I do not have cells available, and my cognitive functioning "floods." Moreover, it is not easy to explain to others that my cognitives are shutting down.

In the last few years, cognitive problems with MS have become recognized. However, it is still not easily discussed; cognition goes to the core of who we are, and often people do not want to acknowledge or even know about it. I have been at MS support group meetings where bladder control and erectile dysfunction are discussed openly and with ease. If I mention cognition, the room goes silent, and no one wants to talk about it.

In addition to acknowledging cognitive loss, I manage this MS symptom with medication, compensatory techniques, and rehabilitation. The medications I tried for cognition had not been studied for MS. However, with my doctor's supervision, I took Aricept and memantine. As for compensatory techniques, the expert advice is not very advanced. The best suggestion that they offer is to keep a "to do" list, something a life-long obsessive-compulsively organized person like me has been doing forever! I also have routines and systems to remind me to take medicines, that I have an appliance working, and how to reorient myself when I get on cognitive overload.

I tried structured cognitive rehabilitation—even going to an Alzheimer's clinic—for many months to see whether their techniques could have application to my MS. Finally, I met with a psychologist who helped me develop rehabilitation techniques. We took certain activities (most of which I was unfamiliar with) and combined them, trying to create new pathways in my brain, retrain and reinforce old pathways, and establish new skills to have as backups to existing pathways. For example, I memorize verses; take piano lessons; do origami, needlepoint, and jigsaw puzzles; play card games; and juggle. As I improve in these functions I try to do these tasks and add in NPR or a recorded book in the background. It is humbling to struggle through things many kindergartners do with ease. It is both frustrating and a bit frightening when I find myself unable to recall how to do the task or to start to "melt down" as I re-re-re-remember the song I played last month on the piano. However, it can also be empowering to finally be able to master turning a piece of paper into a bunny or a series of notes on a page into music.

Recently, my husband came home and said, "What a great origami bird. I think you've got it. I am so proud." At first I shared in this feeling of triumph. Then reality hit, and I gave him a twofold response, "A, this is not a bird: it is a flower, and B, I did not go to law school for 3 years to make paper toys!" Before MS, I was smart with little effort; now it is enough to try to be smart about the loss of my cognitive ability and to do what I can to retain and retrain it.

36. How long will I be able to walk? Will I get paralyzed and end up in a wheelchair?

The ability to walk is affected in an increasing proportion of untreated MS patients over time. However, the rate of progression varies from patient to patient. Frequent attacks with incomplete recovery are indicators of a poorer outlook. Importantly, the likelihood of disability is diminished by (early) therapeutic intervention.

The studies of the natural history of MS in patients in southern Ontario documented that half of those who had three attacks within their first year required the use of wheelchairs within 5 years of onset. In reality, those (untreated) patients will often be wheelchair bound within 2 years. This kind of progression warrants an aggressive approach to MS management.

37. Will I regain my bladder control?

The loss of bladder function occurs in a proportion of patients. With acute attacks when control of voiding is lost, recovery follows promptly. However, from several older studies of patients with long-term follow-up, it is apparent than eventually about two thirds of the patients may be left with some impairment of bladder function.

Expert care of the bladder is important in all patients. Prompt and effective management of infections and measures taken to prevent infections are primary issues. Many urologists are less interested in medical **urology** and lack appropriate diagnostic equipment to

Urology

the field of medical care dealing with diseases of the kidneys bladder and associated structures including the ureters, urethra, etc.

evaluate patients fully. All patients with bladder or kidney infections should have appropriate urine specimens submitted for examination and culture before taking antibiotics. If the organism identified appears resistant to the antibiotic originally prescribed and the patient is not responding to treatment, a more appropriate antibiotic can be selected from the culture report. With effective treatment of infection, the bladder is likely to function more normally than one that is chronically irritated. Drugs that reduce the irritability of the bladder can be helpful but do not replace antibiotics for infections.

PART FOUR

Causes of Multiple Sclerosis

What causes MS?

Do viruses cause MS?

What is the role of the immune system in MS?

Is MS hereditary?

More...

38. What causes MS?

There is no simple single answer to the questions "what causes MS?" or "why do some people get MS?" Over the last century and a half, three important inter-related contributing factors have been recognized: environmental (usually thought to be infectious), immune, and **hereditary** (genetic) factors. Obviously, it would be impossible to do more than superficially discuss these issues. The most commonly asked questions are addressed.

Population studies have yielded information from which it has been inferred that an **environmental factor** exists. Persons moving from high-risk to low-risk areas take the risk with them if they move after the age of 15 years. Conversely, if they move before the age of 15 years, they appear to leave the risk behind. This information comes from studies of populations moving from Europe (a high-risk area) to Africa (a low-risk area). Similar observations have been noted in the populations moving into Israel. These findings, as well as the occurrence of an epidemic of MS in the Faeroe Islands after the "invasion" of those islands by British troupes at the outset of World War II, suggest that an infectious agent is playing a role in MS.

INFECTIONS AND MS

39. Do viruses cause MS?

The onset of an acute demyelinating disease (**postinfectious encephalomyelitis**) occurs after a number of different infections such as measles and mumps as well as smallpox **vaccination**. About one quarter of these cases diagnosed as postinfectious encephalomyelitis

Hereditary

transmitted from parent to child by information contained in the genes.

Environmental factor

any factor in the environment that may contribute to the risk of a disease, such as MS. The environmental factor in MS is assumed to be a virus.

Postinfectious encephalomyelitis

acute disseminated encephalomyelitis occurring following an infection.

Vaccination

the deliberate induction of adaptive immunity to a pathogen by injecting a vaccine, a dead or attenuated (non-pathogenic) form of the pathogen.

end up with a diagnosis of MS. This naturally raised the theory that viruses might be the cause of MS. Over the years, research has implicated many infectious agents, such as the measles virus (and other paramyxoviruses), **distemper**, the **T-cell** leukemia virus, as well as certain **bacteria**, as possible environmental factors. For the most part, they have been discarded. No single infection is known to cause MS.

40. What does herpes (virus) have to do with MS?

The **herpes** families of viruses are DNA viruses that once inside our bodies persist for the rest of our lives. Although herpes simplex type I (HSV-1) and type II (HSV-2) can live in neurons and seem to be protected by them, there is no evidence that they or another family of herpes viruses (**cytomegaloviruses**) have any potential role in the causation or reactivation of MS. Although another herpes virus (the chickenpox or zoster virus) can cause demyelination in rare circumstances, this virus has no demonstrated role in MS. In the last few years, attention has turned to other herpes viruses, specifically the **Epstein-Barr virus** (**EBV**) and herpes simplex virus 6 (HSV-6).

41. My doctor told me that I have antibody to the Epstein-Barr virus. Why do I have this antibody if I have MS?

All of us encounter the EBV at some point in our lives. The very young and the old may not have any

Distemper

illness in dogs and cats caused by the measles like distemper paramyxovirus of the same name.

T-cell

a subset of lymphocytes developing in the thymus. Killer T-cell is the common term for a cytotoxic T-cell.

Bacteria

microscopic infectious organisms that cause a variety of diseases in humans and other species.

Herpes

several species (types) of Herpes virus are responsible for diseases including chickenpox, shingles, mononucleosis, (fever blisters or cold sores and roseola infantum.

Cytomegaloviruses

a family of herpes viruses that inhabit the urinary tract of almost all humans.

Epstein-Barr virus (EBV)

a member of the herpes virus family and one of the most common human viruses.

Causes

symptoms accompanying their infection, but adolescents and young adults characteristically experience marked fatigue and have large **lymph glands** with the infection. Antibody levels in most infected people fall and may seem to disappear over a long period of time. However, many patients with MS have higher than normal levels of antibody (including so-called "early" antibodies to this virus as well as many other viruses and substances). It is generally accepted that this antibody appears to be due to a problem of the immune responses rather than evidence that the Epstein-Barr virus is playing a role in MS. Recently, some scientists have reported that one third of MS patients have virus antibody in their spinal fluid that is not present in others. The importance of this finding is uncertain. Other exciting work has shown immunologic cross-reactivity of MS patient's lymphocytes between EBV and a brain protein, **myelin basic protein**. This means that the human immune system reacting to a protein in the EBV virus can cross-react with a brain protein and produce myelin damage. No final conclusions about these findings have been reached.

42. What is the importance of HSV-6 in MS?

Currently, a great deal of interest is in the newly recognized family of viruses known as HSV-6. This virus family is distantly related to HSV-1 (the cold sore virus) but is very closely related to the EBV and yet another family of viruses called HSV-7. Both HSV-6 and another closely related virus HSV-7 share two thirds of their DNA structure with the EBV virus. Cross-reactivity of antibody to these viruses might be one explanation of the finding of "antibody to EBV" in

Lymph glands

collections of lymphocytes into organs of immune function, also called lymph nodes.

Myelin basic protein

a structural protein of myelin. It is the most potent protein capable of stimulating the immune system.

MS. Both HSV-6 and HSV-7, as well as EBV, can infect the cells of the immune system (lymphocytes) and stimulate them to uncontrolled reproduction (immortalize them). Although all three viruses can infect the immune system and immortalize them, only HSV-6 and HSV-7 can infect cells in the nervous system. The HSV-6 virus has been found in the cells that make myelin, the oligodendrocytes, of MS patients. Research into a possible role for EBV, HSV-6, and other related viruses continues. No convincing relationship of HSV-6 or HSV-7 to MS has, as yet, been firmly established. However, this remains an active and important area of research.

43. Is chlamydia a cause of MS?

Chlamydia pneumoniae and, more recently, *Acinetobacter* are other organisms that have been implicated by other research. The chlamydia (*C. pneumoniae*) that is being studied is not the organism that commonly causes sexually transmitted disease. Although research continues, these agents have not been shown to play any specific role in MS.

IMMUNITY AND MS
44. What is the role of the immune system in MS?

A great deal of evidence has been accumulated over the last several decades that abnormal immune reactions against myelin proteins can be detected in patients with MS. Although antibodies to myelin are common in patients with MS, they are also common in patients with other disorders as well.

Causes

Chlamydia pneumoniae

a bacterium that can cause pneumonia that has been studied as a potential factor in MS as well as other diseases.

Acinetobacter

a bacterium that infects the upper respiratory tract and that has been hypothesized to be a causative factor in MS by some researchers in England.

The occurrence of inflammatory disease of the brain and spinal cord (acute encephalomyelitis) following infections and immunizations (especially after a killed virus rabies vaccine made from rabbit spinal cord) led to studies of the "allergic" potential of certain proteins in the nervous system. Most research has been focused on a single protein, myelin basic protein, because it has a high potential for the induction of experimental demyelinating disease in rats, guinea pigs, monkeys, and other animals. Only 10 millionths of a gram (there are 450 grams in a pound) injected into a genetically susceptible rat can result in experimental disease resembling MS. Over 30 years ago we found that MS patients have cells reactive to this protein in their blood. More recently, Swedish scientists have also found cells with similar reactivity in the spinal fluid of MS patients. Importantly, the original research into a treatment now approved for use in MS (Copaxone) arose from this work. Copaxone is a synthetic "fake" brain protein that serves as a decoy to redirect immune reactions away from myelin basic protein in myelin.

Proteolipid

a structural protein of myelin.

Mutation

a change in the structure of DNA with a potential to alter the normal function of the gene.

Familial infantile spastic paraplegia

a group of different genetic disorders that cause spasticity in family members, usually occurring in infancy.

In recent years, other nervous system proteins have been implicated in autoallergic central nervous system diseases. A large myelin protein (**proteolipid**) has been used to induce experimental disease. A dozen and a half **mutations** (which are changes in the structure of the DNA with the potential to alter the normal function of the gene) of the gene coding for this protein have been found in different families with **familial infantile spastic paraplegia**, a nervous system disease than superficially resembles MS. Despite this advance in understanding of those rare disorders, it does not seem to have any importance in MS. We have found that immune responses to this protein in MS patients are difficult to detect and when found do not occur more commonly than in patients with other nervous system diseases.

Currently, a great deal of interest is being focused on another protein, which has recently been found in miniscule quantities in the central nervous system called **myelin oligodendrocyte glycoprotein (MOG)**. Monkeys immunized with MOG protein have a disease more closely resembling the human disease than disease induced with myelin basic protein. Moreover, in recent unconfirmed studies, antibody to this protein has been reported to be present in the blood of patients with their very first manifestation of illness (MS). This is particularly important because MOG antibody is capable of transferring disease in primates. Antibody to MOG is found in a high proportion of MS patients with progressive disease, also. This finding makes its significance more difficult to understand. Research continues without a firm role for anti-MOG antibody being established. However, there is a suspicion that immune reactions to this protein may be of importance in a subset of patients in whom antibody appears to be playing a central role.

Causes

Myelin oligodendrocyte glycoprotein (MOG)

specific protein found in oligodendrocytes and in myelin.

45. What is autoimmunity?

Autoimmunity is an immune reaction against "self." Autoimmune disease implies that tissue damage is a result of an autoimmune (autoallergic) reaction. This may be the result of antibody production or as a result of lymphocytes (CD4+) causing damage directly or in concert with macrophages. There is a third type of immunologic reaction, an antibody-mediated tissue damage in which different lymphocytes (CD8+) cause additional damage. All three types of reactions are

Autoimmunity

The consequence of the arousal of the immune system leading to antibody production or a cellular (lymphocyte) reaction directed against tissues in ones own body (antigens).

thought to play a role in some patients with MS. Recent evidence implicates CD8+ cells in attacks of demyelinating disease called acute disseminated encephalomyelitis that, although resembling MS, does not relapse. It is like a "single attack of MS" type of disease.

46. Do antibodies cause MS?

For a long time, antibody was considered to be a likely cause of myelin damage in MS, but the theory fell into disrepute. More recently, there appears to be stronger evidence that an antibody to a newly recognized myelin protein (anti-MOG antibody) may be playing a role in some patients. Additional evidence comes from analysis of brain tissue from patients in whom antibody has been deposited on myelin and an antibody-mediated, CD8+ lymphocyte type of **pathology** is present. It is not known whether this antibody is truly anti-MOG, but as described previously here, anti-MOG antibody was recently detected in the blood of patients at the very outset of their illness. Other studies have shown that a high proportion of patients with progressive illness also have this antibody in their blood. However, this does not necessarily mean that the antibody is causing the myelin damage.

Pathology

the scientific study of disease. It is also a term used to describe detectable damage to tissues.

47. What causes an MS plaque?

The typical MS plaque seen in patients who have died early in their illness or who have had brain biopsies is composed of a mixture of lymphocytes with many more macrophages, without antibody. The macrophages in the plaque contain myelin within their cell bodies in various stages of digestion. Some axons are damaged, but they are relatively preserved as compared with myelin. After the initial insult by these cells, scarring begins. This process varies greatly from one individual to another. Curiously, the macrophages contain hormones like **brain-derived nerve growth factor** that should stimulate repair. The macrophage also secretes another hormone that stimulates scarring (**T-cell growth factor beta-1**). The invading cells seeking to remove some unknown enemy virus or protein seem prepared to help in rebuilding the damaged tissue. Later in the development of the plaque, scarring occurs. It is this scarring that makes the plaque hard (**sclerotic**). In summary, the plaque is an area of intense inflammation with myelin damage where the nerve fibers are relatively preserved and show variable amounts of scarring.

48. Is there a connection between virus infection and autoimmune disease?

A comment about the relationship of virus infection to autoimmune disease in general is warranted. **Infectious mononucleosis** occurs only when adolescents or young adults are infected with the EBV. The symptoms of infectious mononucleosis (and other autoimmune phenomena) occur as a result of the immune reaction to the viral infection. Dr. Gertrude Henle, who discovered the relationship between EBV and infectious mononucleosis, studied a possible link between MS and this virus; it was concluded that there was none. Research continues because of consistently high antibody titers to EBV in many patients with MS. HSV-6 and HSV-7 are very closely related families of viruses. Indeed, their structure (EBV, HSV-6, and HSV-7) is two thirds identical, which has made

Brain-derived nerve growth factor
a specific nervous system hormone which can stimulate repair of the nervous system.

T-cell growth factor beta-1
an interleukin (hormone) produced by lymphocytes that stimulates scarring in tissues. It also stimulates myelin formation.

Sclerotic
a term referring to hardened tissue such as MS plaques in the brain. This hardness or sclerosis is caused by scarring.

Infectious mononucleosis
glandular fever. It is a common form of infection with the Epstein-Barr virus (EBV) consisting of fever, fatigue, enlarged lymph nodes, often with rash, splenic enlargement and hepatic enzyme elevation.

Causes

progress difficult. An immune reaction to tissue damaged by an immune reaction has been theorized to cause damage to myelin as well as other tissues. There is now good evidence in experimental animals and in humans that this is correct. Another theory is that part of the protein in a virus is similar in some aspect or even identical to a natural protein in myelin or other tissue. As noted previously, an immune reaction to seemingly dissimilar proteins, one being a myelin protein and the other a component of the EBV, has been documented. An immune response to the virus can result in myelin damage. Regulation or control of immune responses may be genetically impaired to a greater or lesser degree in certain patients.

In summary, it is theorized that a virus that children are protected from early in life infects genetically predisposed adolescents. This results in an immune reaction to proteins in the virus that resemble proteins in myelin, thus initiating an attack of the person's own myelin in MS. This immune attack then leads to additional damage to myelin (and other nervous system tissue). The damage to normal tissues is then followed by additional immune reactions and more potential attacks. Immunologists think that part of the problem is an ineffective control of the immune reaction in MS patients that allows additional attacks to occur.

GENETICS AND MS
49. Is MS hereditary?

Genetic factors are recognized as playing a role in MS. *This is not to say that they cause MS.* Although MS is typically a disease of people of European ancestry, it also occurs in African Americans, who share genes common in both African and European populations. The observation that MS is about one half as common in African Americans as white Americans would seem to correlate with a risk related to European ancestry. Among Europeans, MS is much more common in northwestern Europe, particularly in Scandinavia, Scotland, and Ireland. However, as physicians trained in neurology returned to areas in southern Europe that were considered to be low-risk areas, such as Sardinia and Sicily, MS became diagnosed much more often. Indeed, these two areas are now considered to be high-risk areas. These observations have been interpreted to suggest that hereditary factors as well as environmental factors are involved in the risk of MS.

Certain specific genes are more common in MS patient populations. Each of the genes HLA-A3, HLA-B7, and DR-2 (now often referred to DR-1 1501b), which are all located on **chromosome** six, are each twice as common in MS as compared with the general population. However, the majority of persons in those populations with these genes do not have MS, clearly indicating that they are not "MS genes." Ten years ago, the DR gene was proven to be an immune response gene. DR-2 is simply a genetic mutation of the immune response gene that is twice as common in the MS population as compared with the general population. DR-2 is now more correctly identified as DR-1 1501b. It is possible that certain mutations of immune response genes are more efficient in their function in turning on immune responses, as least as far as reactions to nervous system proteins. MS is not a simple hereditary disease, but it does appear more commonly in families of MS patients.

Chromosome
genetic material collected in the nucleus within each cell.

Karen's comment:

My two sisters and I are often mistaken for triplets. We have statistically the least likely genetic composition that could result from our parents. Our tall, dark brown-eyed, brunette mother often called the three of us short, blue-eyed, blond daughters her "recessives!" My youngest sister has two daughters who also resemble us. There is a lot of immune-based illness in our family, including diabetes and allergy. When one sister had a ringing in her ear and migraines and a niece had unexplained falls, we held our collective breath until MS was ruled out for each of them. So far, I am the only one in my family who has been diagnosed with MS; however, I qualify this with "so far," as it is a concern that we cannot ignore.

50. Will my children get MS?

Children of parents with MS have an increased risk of developing MS. The chance is relatively small, however. Many years ago, studies in Minnesota established that the risk for children born to a mother with MS is 20 to 40 times higher than for the general population and that female children have twice the risk as males. However, these children will be under greater surveillance than the general population, and a diagnosis of MS is less likely to be missed. Parents and other family members are not likely to ignore symptoms of milder illness. The risk in the general population is quite small, and even at such elevated risks, this corresponds to small percentages.

Recent studies in Canada suggest that parents with the "DR-2" gene (DR1 1501b) have an even higher risk of transmitting the probability of MS to their children than had been thought previously. It is clear from these studies that mothers have the greatest risk of passing on an increased risk of MS to their children, with girls possessing the "DR-2" gene having the greatest risk. Care must be taken before extrapolating these observations to other populations, however. For example, we have found that DR-2 is rare in the Cuban American population, but MS is relatively common in this population. The population of patients with MS in Sardinia has been studied intensively, and they, too, appear to have different genes that correlate with their risk of MS. Siblings are reportedly 10 times more likely to develop MS than the general population. It is probably more correct to say that their risk of being diagnosed is 10 to 20 times greater.

51. What are genes? What genes cause MS?

Genes are the smallest bits of DNA that can pass on a hereditary characteristic to a child. They are located almost exclusively in chromosomes that are contained in the **nucleus** in the center of every cell in the body. Genes related to energy production are present in the **mitochondria**. Mutations are changes in the structure of the DNA that often alter the normal function of that gene. For those readers interested in the details of genes and their function, reviews of the subject can be found in the *Scientific American* and encyclopedias.

Although there are probably no "MS genes" as such, MS patients have certain genes more commonly than other people. The best known of these genes that occur more often in MS are members of the major histocompatibility loci (MHC) located on chromosome 6

Nucleus
the cellular organelle enclosing the chromosomes. It is bounded by a nuclear membrane.

Mitochondria
the cells' power sources. They usually are rod-shaped but can be round. They have an outer membrane that limits the organelle and an inner membrane thrown into folds projecting inwards.

(Figure 7) at a point on the short arm of the chromosome at location number 21. You have probably heard of these in relationship to organ transplantation but the majority of genes that play a role in immune function and autoimmunity are located in this location. There are 4 of these important gene loci (locations), A, B, C, and D. The "A" locus is a gene that codes for the MHC "class I protein" and it is the actual immune response gene for antibody production. The "DR" gene (at the D locus) is another immune response gene that codes for the so-called "MHC class II protein" that plays a central role in cell-mediated immunity. These reactions principally involve monocytes and CD4 lymphocytes. Although, the B locus is near the D locus, its role is obscure. There are many additional genes in this region of chromosome 6 that are involved in immune reactions.

Mutations have occurred at a higher rate in the MHC region than in the rest of the human genome. Several mutations or alterations in this region that are more common in MS have been identified. These are sometimes referred to as **polymorphisms**. As you have undoubtedly heard the human genome project has deciphered our genetic code but many details regarding genes remain to be discovered. The human genome project is presently looking for a pattern of **single nucleotide polymorphisms** (SNPs [pronounced as *snips*]) (i.e., a "signature group of gene alterations" in MS). Once an individual SNP is identified a search for the identity and function of the actual gene follows. A number of SNPs are anticipated to be associated with a predisposition to MS, as has been established for **Crohn's disease**, another autoimmune illness. Separately, in a recent Swedish study funded by the Montel Williams Foundation, the MHC2TA gene

Polymorphisms

referring to genetic polymorphisms, meaning many forms or shapes indicating the presence of mutations, chromosomal breaks, and transpositions, etc.

Single Nucleotide polymorphisms (SNPs)

a group of gene alterations that may be a "signature group" for a disease.

Crohn's disease

an autoimmune inflammatory disease of bowel principally, but not exclusively, affecting small bowel. It occurs with increased frequency in MS patients.

(a "transactivator" gene at the MHC region) has been shown to be associated with increased susceptibility to MS and rheumatoid arthritis. The identification of specific genes predisposing to MS hopefully will lead to preventative strategies.

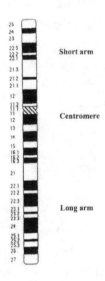

Figure 7. Drawing of chromosome 6 from the Human Genome Project. This drawing represents one of the pair of chromosomes. A chromosome has two arms or telomeres, a short arm and a long arm. There is a numbering system which starts at the centromere, the place where the telomeres join. Note the short arm (above) and also note position 21. This region (21) contains the "major histocompatibility (MHC)" genes. HLA-A, HLA-B, and DR. Many genes concerned with immune function are present in this region of chromosome 6. Collectively, genes of this part of the human genome have the highest rate of genetic mutation compared with any other part.

52. Is there a genetic reason why some people have severe disease?

In all probability, there is a genetic reason for a very small percentage of patients having very severe disease. Thirty-five years ago, a Danish group in Copenhagen found that when they tested MS patients who had suffered this rapidly progressive malignant disease, the majority of them had both the B-7 and DR-2 genes. It is now known that the gene for **tumor necrosis factor**, which is a principal factor in damaging myelin, is contained within this region and that there are more active mutations of these genes in some MS patients than in normal individuals. The extension of the human genome project, it is hoped, will extend these findings and shed further light on these genetic associations with severe disease. New specific therapeutic interventions may then follow.

Tumor necrosis factor

a principal factor made by macrophages that damage myelin.

OTHER FACTORS

53. I read that toxins can cause MS. Is this true? Can I be detoxified?

When people thought about toxins in the past, they usually referred to mercury, lead, arsenic, antimony, and other metals. Nowadays, insecticides are more often considered as potentially injurious. Hydrocarbons, poly-chlor-vinyls (PCVs) used in the manufacture of certain plastics, and other organic compounds are also topics of conversation and speculation regarding their impact on myelin and nervous system disease in general.

In fact, many potential toxins exist in our environment, but federal agencies and groups within our society are making progress in reducing exposure to these agents. Problems caused by lead, mercury, and arsenic are real but do not appear to be issues that are especially relevant to MS patients. Few facts are available as to how much these toxins affect normal persons in the concentrations encountered in the environment, let alone how they may impact patients with MS. There is indeed more myth than fact regarding the role of toxins in health and disease.

One continuing concern is whether mercury in **dental amalgam**, the material used in dental fillings, is a health issue for MS. Although industrial mercury pollution was a major health problem in Japan and elsewhere, mercury in dental amalgam is a very different issue. There are inconsequential differences in serum and tissue levels of mercury in MS patients as compared with normals. We have found no differences in urinary excretion of mercury in MS patients. In studies of edentulous MS patients who had never had any dental repairs, we found they had higher levels of mercury simply because they consumed more fish. Thus, there is no medical justification for removal of amalgam dental fillings, and the concept of "detoxification" has no place in the management of MS. Increased excretion of metals after "chelation" with drugs does not mean toxic levels were present in the person prior to chelation. Many of the measurements reported by laboratories are unreliable. Hair analysis is preferred, but hair from the head is not suitable. Slow growing hair such as pubic hair is the only appropriate specimen. Most patients, and some physicians, are unaware that chelating agents are themselves quite toxic and should be avoided, especially in treating MS patients! The bottom line is that there is no role for chelation therapy in MS.

Dental amalgam
the material dentists used for dental repairs (make dental fillings).

Causes

54. Why do veterans have more MS?

The epidemiologic analysis of veterans' records for MS was not based on any evidence that veterans had an increased risk of MS, nor has any been accumulated that military service increases the risk of MS. Certainly, there are abundant data showing that stress impacts health in a variety of ways. Stress may be a factor in precipitating MS in the same ways in military life as in civilian life. However, the subject of military service, exposure to toxins peculiar to military life, and an increased risk of MS have not been the specific aim of any prospective studies.

55. Can stress cause MS?

Stress has been shown to be an aggravating factor in MS but not a causal factor. More than 30 years ago, in conjunction with the McGill department of psychiatry in Montreal, we found that major life stress (such as death or serious illness in a child or other family member, marital discord, and loss of employment) was three to four times more common in MS patients than in medical patients who had been referred to psychiatrists for psychiatric consultation and care. Moreover, this stress was temporarily associated with relapses. We also found that major life stress was two to three times more common in the medical patients requiring psychiatric care than those not in need of psychiatric help.

Our finding that there is an association between stressful life events and attacks of MS has been confirmed and extended in a number of studies in the United States and Canada. The most impressive was a San Francisco study showing that MS patients have new brain lesions detected in MRI brain scans more frequently when confronted with acute stress. A surprising finding was that "hassles," those more minor irritations that just won't go away, were also associated with an increased risk of new brain lesions.

Certainly, there is a need for further scientific study of the biological consequences of stress and autoimmune disease. Such studies could lead to useful therapeutic interventions.

56. Can accidents bring on attacks of MS?

There is relevant history behind the issue of trauma and the risk of attacks, or the onset, of MS. The great Dr. Douglas McAlpine achieved international recognition for his specialization in MS at the Middlesex Hospital in London. Among his many original observations, he was the first to recognize that physical trauma increased the risk of MS exacerbations.

After moving to Montreal from Boston in 1971, I had the good fortune to work with my esteemed colleague, J. Bertrand R. (Bert) Cosgrove, at the Montreal Neurological Institute (the "MNI"), at McGill University. He had been trained in neurology at the National Hospital at Queen Square in London (England) and with Dr. McAlpine. At that time, I was introduced to the reality of the clinical problem of MS.

We saw large numbers of MS patients, and Dr. Cosgrove introduced me to a myriad of less commonly recognized issues that patients with this disease confront. Dr. Cosgrove was especially interested and introduced me to the issue of factors that increase the risk of exacerbations of MS. He pointed out that these factors included pregnancy, infection, burns, electric shock, stress, and surgical or accidental trauma.

Dr. Cosgrove emphasized that trauma, whatever the cause, was inevitably associated with emotional stress. With Dr. Lucien Gratton, a French psychopharmacologist, we prospectively studied stress and found a strong association between stress and new attacks of MS. Dr. Cosgrove attributed the first recognition of these aggravating factors to Dr. McAlpine.

Despite the observations of McAlpine and Cosgrove, the relationship between trauma and onset or worsening of MS is considered to be unproven by some. Physicians of limited experience particularly echo this. However, critics are correct when they point out that this has not been studied scientifically. In the original observations, McAlpine did review his detailed clinical records retrospectively and did report a doubling of the risk of an attack of MS in association with surgery or other trauma. He pointed out that this appeared to be true even for dental extraction. In fairness, McAlpine's records were recorded and collected prospectively and in a more modern sense were a database recorded on paper.

Dr. Cosgrove, however, observed that certain traumas were associated with greater risk than others. Importantly, accidents and surgical trauma similarly are associated with psychologic stress. It is difficult, in most situations, therefore, to separate the physical from the psychologic component in accidents and their individual contributions in this regard. If this is true, how can it be explained? Tissue trauma necessarily activates the immune system, which might reasonably lead to an increased risk of an attack of autoimmune disease *in genetically predisposed individuals.* It is likely that this reaction might serve to make a minor attack more clinically apparent.

Causes

PART FIVE

Living with

Multiple Sclerosis

Now that I have been diagnosed with MS, how do I learn to cope with this disease?

What do I need to know now that I have been diagnosed with MS?

So many people want to be helpful, but I'm feeling overwhelmed and am not sure whether the information I am getting is correct. Where should I go for help?

More...

57. Now that I have been diagnosed with MS, how do I learn to cope with this disease?

Over the last four decades that I have dealt with persons diagnosed with MS, I have learned that each person reacts somewhat differently to a new diagnosis of MS. In many patients, the diagnosis is welcomed as an explanation for an event affecting their health that had previously remained unexplained. Others anticipated the diagnosis on the basis of life experience (the experience of a friend, relative, or celebrity dealing with MS). In some, surfing the web or reading provided some insight into the illness. However, many come to MS centers for a "second opinion" because of an uncertain prior diagnosis.

The first step in dealing with MS is acceptance of the diagnosis (i.e., what does the diagnosis mean?). A diagnosis may be easy for the neurologist, but the affected person may not react positively or may even be suspicious about the seeming ease of establishing the diagnosis. Obviously, the confidence in the physician is a prerequisite in accepting the diagnosis. Although physicians other than neurologists may suspect the diagnosis, *the diagnosis of MS must be made by a neurologist.* It is also assumed that appropriate clinical neurologic examinations and tests such as MRIs of the brain and spinal cord, cerebrospinal fluid (CSF) examination, and certain blood work will be performed and the results reviewed. These tests are usually needed to eliminate other diseases. Illnesses that can sometimes mimic MS, such as **syphilis, system lupus erythematosus (SLE)**, and vitamin B12 deficiency, must be eliminated from consideration. Occasionally, patients will have MS as well as another disorder. One of the

Syphilis

an infection due to Treponema pallidum. These infections are similar in type to infections by tuberculosis but are potentially more serious.

System lupus erythematosus (SLE)

a chronic autoimmune disorder that may affect many organ systems including the skin, joints and internal organs. The disease may be mild or severe and life-threatening.

most common additional conditions found in MS is **hypothyroidism**.

An important practical point is that until the patient readily accepts the diagnosis any decision regarding therapy has to be considered a tentative or a temporary decision. The evidence is clear that *early treatment in MS is more effective,* and withdrawal of treatment may seem to precipitate additional (rebound) attacks in some people. Despite the importance of initiating treatment, some patients cannot readily accept the diagnosis and need assistance in dealing with the realities of their disease. The classic book *Denial of Illness* was based on the author's (Dr. Weinstein) experience with MS patients in a New York City MS clinic. It was the difficulty of MS patients in accepting the diagnosis and the implications of such a diagnosis that led to his classic publication. Denial of illness is not uncommon in young adults, but it seems to be seen disproportionately more often in persons with MS.

A patient may accept the authority of the diagnosing neurologist without question, but in these times, this is somewhat unusual. It is important that patients who are faced with the pronouncement of the diagnosis of MS are able to discuss the basis of the diagnosis and communicate with their neurologist. Most patients ask the questions posed in Part I, such this: "What is MS?" These are real questions asked by real people. Although we know a great deal about the disease process in MS, we do not know the cause of MS (any more than we know the cause of cancer). However, in today's world, every new treatment is based on theories of how drugs interact with one or more steps in the disease process in MS. The results of these trials, regardless of a positive or negative outcome, provide

Hypothyroidism
a disease of the thyroid associated with decreased secretion of thyroid hormone.

Living with Multiple Sclerosis

new and better understanding of MS. With the great progress that has been made in the last 10 years, I anticipate that clarification of each step of the pathogenesis of the disease process will be accomplished and accepted in the near future.

58. What do I need to know now that I have been diagnosed with MS?

You do not need to know how to make a watch to read time. In other words, it is not so important to understand every aspect of the MS disease process as it is to know that the vast majority of patients with MS will have the disease throughout their lifetime. Patients with MS will almost certainly have new symptoms along with relapses of old symptoms, with attacks tending to decrease in frequency and severity over the years. The interval between these attacks cannot be predicted with any accuracy, but most MS patients have an attack frequency ranging from one attack in 4 years to two or more each year. For some patients, there is a tendency over a period of time to develop some disability. This is more serious when disability progresses between attacks and is the basis for making a diagnosis of secondary progressive disease (discussed in Part Three). A recently published study of the natural course of MS in patients at the Mayo Clinic found that, on average, no statistically significant progression of disability occurred over a period of 10 years! However, 30% of the patients did experience progression of disability. This kind of information is important to consider in making therapeutic decisions. Importantly, a variety of treatments for MS have been shown to have an impact on virtually every type of disease that we recognize as MS (Part Six).

59. So many people want to be helpful, but I'm feeling overwhelmed and am not sure whether the information I am getting is correct. Where should I go for help?

The understanding, experienced physician is sufficient to meet the needs of most patients with MS. Often it is a matter of sweeping away unfounded fears and false conclusions about the disease and the effect of the disease on function. Friends and families are important to patients and often provide wonderful support. However, the information that they have is not always correct or reasonably up-to-date.

Physicians encounter patients (and sometimes their immediate family members) who when coached to ask appropriate questions spill out baseless perceptions that severe disability such as paralysis and sexual dysfunction occurs often and early in their illness. Each of us has our own particular set of fears when it comes to how an illness will impact us. Doctors and nurses are no exceptions.

60. I'm having trouble coping with this diagnosis. Should I seek professional counseling?

When faced with stress, it is difficult for us to understand and accept difficult issues such as a new diagnosis. Psychological counseling may help some patients with anxiety resulting from the stress related to their diagnosis. The inability to predict the course of MS, apart from a few generalities regarding the illness, sometimes detracts from any confidence the patients might have in the treating neurologist. No neurologist can foretell the course for an individual patient, but MS takes on certain predictabilities in relationship to the course of illness, as outlined briefly in the previous paragraph. The reality of predictably effective, safe, and convenient therapy promises to take out much of the sting associated with accepting the diagnosis of MS. However, some will require the help of social workers, psychologists, or even psychiatrists to help them cope with anxiety precipitated by the new diagnosis.

61. Are there any MS "groups" that I can look into for additional help?

The National Multiple Sclerosis Society (NMSS) chapters and other groups have played an important part in education of patients and their families about MS. The MS Society chapters have regularly supported educational lectures for MS patients and their families. These sessions sometimes double as group therapy. When supervised by a professional, they are of real value to participants. Certainly, meeting other patients and exchanging experiences can help put the disease in perspective. It is important to recognize that the clinical course of illness varies greatly from one person to another. Young people may be intimidated when they meet severely affected individuals, regardless of the age or duration of illness. Therefore, potential participants in these sessions may wish to get more information about who will be present at a particular group session they are considering attending and whether it will be led by a knowledgeable professional.

The NMSS prints many helpful brochures, but the practice of mailing out dozens of brochures to unsuspecting newly diagnosed patients can be intimidating and, of course, wasteful.

Karen's comment:

I am not drawn to groups; usually I prefer a talk with God, a close friend, or a family member as a source of support. Nevertheless, I participate in MS support groups. I find them to be helpful as sources of information, and I hope I have been a source of support for other people. As with any group, there are dynamics and politics.

MS as a common bond makes it no more or less likely that I will necessarily like or want to spend time with a person. However, MS has created a connection with and introduced me to people I might never have known otherwise.

The people at the meetings by and large are there for positive reasons. They are generally well informed and well meaning. Additionally, there are the usual characters: the newly diagnosed person in denial who is sure it was a misdiagnosis and expects never to be at another meeting; the recently diagnosed person who expressed the same denial at a prior meeting; the person who is certain of and has all of the answers; the bee sting aficionado; the lonely soul who has no other social contact; the nervous caregiver who eats cookies nonstop; and me. All of these people come together with stories that are unique, unnerving, empowering, irritating, enlightening, heartbreaking, tiring, and fascinating.

MS AND SEXUALITY

62. How does MS affect sexual function?

Patients and physicians in the past rarely discussed sexual function and performance despite its central role in life. This was especially true when illness other than heart disease was at issue. Sexual relationships are a major bond between married couples, and the new frankness about these issues promises to benefit particularly MS patients greatly. There are a number of pertinent issues in this regard, many of which are equally important to healthy persons.

Libido

sexual interest or drive.

The most common sexual problem affecting both men and women in good health is the lack of **libido** (sexual interest or sexual drive). Psychologic stress arising from interpersonal relationships and work is probably the most common single cause for this; it is obviously much more of an issue in young adults affected by a major health problem. The resultant uncertainties that naturally arise in these situations contribute to this greatly. The actual diagnosis of illness may induce acute stress, which can precipitate sexual difficulty or aggravate a pre-existing sexual problem. In both men and women with MS, the loss of a feeling of well-being contributes to sexual dysfunction, whether accompanied by a depressed mood or not. Studies have shown that a caring, understanding relationship between the sexual partners is the single most important factor in maintaining good sexual health. It is important to be aware that the use of drugs for erectile dysfunction does not increase libido. Decision making in regard to changes of lifestyle and treatment for MS is an obviously important issue. Professional counseling is sometimes advisable.

Fatigue is a major symptom in MS and contributes to sexual dysfunction, as it does in healthy men and women. Modification of lifestyle to conserve energy and the use of amantadine or other medications to increase energy are helpful. Amphetamine ("speed"), Ritalin, and cocaine are dangerous and should not be considered. Patients should be cautious of the plethora of products flooding the health food market because some of these agents could actually contain harmful ingredients.

Karen's comment:

The topic of sex and MS has different components: how I feel about myself; how my husband feels about me; and how we feel together. These components naturally intertwine and interact. Before my diagnosis I did not give my body much thought. I felt vibrant and was physically and sexually active, but my sense of myself was more cerebrally focused. I took my body, including sexuality, for granted, assuming that it would all just work without effort or intention. With my diagnosis and the effects of the steroids, I became almost fearful of my body—what was it going to do next? With time, fearless physical therapists, and the love of my husband, I have come to value and work hard on functioning physically. Furthermore, my view of myself sexually is independent of whether all of the parts of my body work on command and without pain. Rather, it depends on how I feel about myself, mind and body.

In the sixth grade, my husband wrote in my autograph book, "Have a great summer and please wear your sexy pink sweater often next year!" After 25 years of marriage he still finds me sexually desirable; when I get out of the shower, he whistles. Nonetheless, MS has had an effect on how he relates to me sexually. Over the years, he has voiced concerns that he could hurt me, worries that I will get tired, and wonders whether I have physical sensations. Together, we manage MS and sex like other issues—with talking, laughing, and crying.

Recently, I was on a panel about issues of illness and care-givers. I relayed our feelings that we do not want my husband to be my full-time caregiver if we can find other good people to help me. Certainly my husband does many care-giving tasks he had not done before my MS. Although he is trained to touch me to help with pain, stiffness, or spasms, we distinguish this "medicinal touch" from sexual touch. Both are done with love but have different mental and physical basis. Not only do we prefer for him not to do certain caregiving functions, he is, by his own admission, much better at taking my clothes off than putting them on. He is totally inept at mascara, and pantyhose get him side-tracked! After I relayed this information to the audience, a petite grandmotherly woman raised her hand to speak: Dr. Ruth gave us her approval!

63. Does Viagra help with impotence in MS?

The physical problem of erectile dysfunction is now openly discussed and is recognized commonly in otherwise healthy men. This change in the public attitude has helped men with MS accept this aspect of sexual function when it occurs and embrace the use of one of the approved drugs for erectile dysfunction. Viagra, Levitra, and Cialis appear to be at least as useful in men with MS as they are in otherwise normal men. Some studies have suggested that these drugs may also be helpful in women having difficulty achieving an **orgasm**. In any case, these medications should be used

Orgasm

Sexual climax.

only under the supervision of a physician. Options other than those just mentioned include drugs inserted into the **urethra** or injected directly into the penis, as well as implantable devices for males not responding to use of these medications. Such issues should be thoroughly discussed with physicians experienced with their use. However, surgery has special risks for men with MS.

Physical limitations affect men more than women in the sex act. The female partner can often compensate for movement difficulties if they limit sexual performance in men. A willingness to experiment is healthy.

64. Are there treatments for loss of genital sensation?

A loss of sensation in the genital area can pose problems for both men and women with MS. Fortunately, such a loss of sensation in most patients is usually temporary. In men, the use of Viagra and the other drugs in this group can, in part, overcome erectile dysfunction related to decreased sensation in some cases. Temporary or not, for many women, the use of vibrators can overcome the inability to achieve orgasm. Eros is a specially designed commercially available device to enhance **clitoral engorgement** and provide stimulation for women who require it. It is important that women consult physicians who are knowledgeable in this area. Generally, **gynecologists** and sex therapists are better informed than most physicians.

Urethra

the anatomical tube connecting the bladder with the outside of the body. In the male it extends to the opening in the penis.

Clitoral engorgement

blood flow to the female sexual organ, the clitoris, is associated with sexual excitement and results in clitoral enlargement (engorgement), and ultimately improves arousal and orgasm (sexual climax) in women.

Gynecologists

physicians who specialize in diseases that uniquely affect women.

Living with Multiple Sclerosis

65. How can I get my wife pregnant if I am impotent?

Semen

the fluid portion of the ejaculate consisting of secretions from the seminal vesicles, prostate gland, and several other glands in the male reproductive tract. Semen may also refer to the entire ejaculate, including the sperm.

Clinics dealing with spinal cord injuries, such as VA hospitals, are able to help with this problem. By using techniques that are similar to those used in animal husbandry, **semen** can be harvested for successful use in **artificial insemination**. Personnel in spinal cord units at VA hospitals and universities should be contacted for help in this regard.

Artificial insemination

achieving pregnancy by artificial means; most commonly semen from a male donor is injected mechanically into the woman's vagina and or uterus.

66. Can pregnancy bring on MS? What are the chances of an attack during pregnancy? Is it true that attacks are more severe after delivery?

Generally, women with MS feel better during pregnancy and have less likelihood of exacerbations of illness. Recent observations reveal that during the first trimester of pregnancy, the rate of attacks may be slightly increased, but during the second trimester, there is a marked lowering of the risk of attack. However, the third trimester is associated with a rising risk of exacerbation. In the 3 months after delivery, the risk is also high. A large French study showed that after delivery of the baby, the risk was increased by a factor of three for the first 3 months postpartum. Unexpectedly, the risk of exacerbations falls somewhat to a twofold risk for the next 33 months.

Earlier smaller studies in Minnesota had revealed an increased propensity to have exacerbations following pregnancy, whether or not the pregnancy went to term (lasted a full 9 months). In other words, termination of the pregnancy does not prevent the likelihood of increased risk of exacerbation and worsened illness.

In summary, the chances of an MS attack during the first trimester of pregnancy are only slightly increased and fall substantially during the second trimester. However, there is an approximately 30% increased likelihood of an exacerbation in the third trimester of pregnancy and a marked increase in the 3 months after delivery. The numbers translate roughly into a 70% chance of exacerbation occurring in the 3-month post delivery period.

Attacks postpartum tend to be more severe than average, but as at other times, the majority of MS attacks are not disabling. Treatment certainly can shorten attacks. The advent of the new and more rapidly effective treatment, natalizumab (Tysabri formerly referred to as Antegren), held the promise of reducing this risk, but this drug has, at least temporarily, been withdrawn from the market. The full effect of natalizumab in preventing attacks of MS is seen within 6 weeks after receiving the first dose. If this drug becomes available, it should not be given to the mother who is breast feeding because of its presence in breast milk; its possible impact on the child has not been studied.

Karen's comment:

I have had many miscarriages and have no children. Before I was diagnosed with MS, I thought I felt good during pregnancy because of emotions of joy and anticipation, and badly after a miscarriage, again because of emotions, albeit ones of grief and loss. Although emotions certainly played a part, I now understand that, as is often the case with MS, I had flare-ups after pregnancy.

Currently, I take estrogen replacement therapy. I am fortunate to have an endocrinologist who is intelligent and who listens to patients. When I began HRT, he informed me about the many estrogens and progesterones. Finding a balance was trial and error—error meant pimples and a desire to murder. The mere mention of the name of one estrogen still strikes terror in my husband!

67. Can pregnancy in a woman with MS harm the unborn child?

There is speculation that fertility is reduced in patients with MS and that the rate of spontaneous abortion is increased in the first trimester of pregnancy. There is no evidence or expectation that MS directly affects the unborn child. However, from the information collected in the North American Research Committee on Multiple Sclerosis (NARCOMS) database, the interferon-beta treatments for MS (Betaseron, Avonex, and Rebif) do pose an increased risk of birth defects in the unborn child.

The increased risk of MS in the child is another issue that has already been discussed. This is a genetic issue and is unrelated to whether the mother was diagnosed prior to the pregnancy.

PART SIX

Treatment

What are the treatments for MS?

Do "folk remedies" such as snake venom and bee venom treatments work?

Is there anything I can do about my overwhelming fatigue?

More...

68. What are the treatments for MS?

Treatment for MS may be divided into three different categories: symptomatic treatment, relapse management, and treatment aimed at the reduction of the risk of relapses as well as disability.

Symptomatic treatment does not alter the disease process but is aimed at relieving symptoms. Treatment of relapses will usually reduce symptoms and the resultant disability associated with the relapse more quickly than would occur naturally, but it does not alter the disease process either. A reduction of relapses will, of course, reduce temporary disability associated with attacks but is most meaningful if it reduces the risk of disability.

Narcotics
derived from the Greek word for stupor, that originally referred to a variety of substances that dulled the senses and relieved pain.

Epilepsy
a brain disorder that occurs when the electrical signals in the brain are disrupted leading to a seizure. People with epilepsy have repeated seizures.

Spasticity
velocity-dependent increase in muscle tone.

Fatigue and urinary tract complaints are among the most common symptoms that MS patients may experience that are amenable to treatment. Many disturbances of sensation are highly subjective symptoms. Not uncommonly, a feeling of numbness is present only when attention is focused on the particular complaint, and it does not interfere with daily activity. Painful sensations may be favorably affected by treatment. Generally, the more severe the pain, the more likely it will be alleviated by medication.

Narcotics are not indicated. Drugs used in the management of **epilepsy** are the mainstay of pain management in MS, although other drugs may also be helpful. The manifestations of **spasticity**, such as stiffness and muscle spasms, can be greatly benefited by treatment.

69. Do "folk remedies" such as snake venom and bee venom treatments work?

Sir Augustus D'Este, a grandson of King George III of England, was the first person clearly known to have MS. The treatment he received, as revealed in his diary, was entirely symptomatic. We would not consider repeated **enemas** and bloodletting to be symptomatic treatment today. Unfortunately, many of the kinds of treatment that today's patients and their families embrace are just as rational as those that he received.

MS treatment in the past was essentially symptomatic —that is, treatment aimed solely at alleviating specific symptoms or making patients feel better. Although that may be good, it is not enough by itself. Treatments were not based on scientific study. Most were not effective, and some were harmful. Today's operators of health food stores sell a large variety of unproven herbal remedies that they justify with unsubstantiated claims. By and large, herbal preparations and most of the preparations sold in such stores should be avoided.

Decades ago, as an intern, I was asked to start IV alcohol on a patient with MS. The prescribing neurosurgeon stated that he had just read a paper in a medical journal claiming benefit for this form of treatment. Despite reservations, I complied. The patient became intoxicated but, nevertheless, felt that she had been helped. The neurosurgeon was embarrassed and abandoned this therapy. Later in my training, I was advised by Lord Brain, a famous British neurologist of the day, that "any drug that had been used for any therapeutic purpose had been tried on patients with MS." I have

Enemas

liquids used to facilitate bowel evacuation; usually water or oil based materials. They are put into the rectum via an enema tube attached to a bag or other container.

Treatment

subsequently come to realize that he was not exaggerating. The major problem is not so much that they are unhelpful but that many treatments are potentially dangerous. Untested drugs, whether purified or in their crude state, should be viewed as potentially dangerous in their own right or by virtue of drug interactions.

Snake Venom

Several decades ago, a self-styled microbiologist in Florida presumed that if an animal (or human) recovered from a snake bite, that recovery occurred because of a biological reaction (perhaps an antibody) that eliminated the offending venom. He reasoned further that the response to snake venom (an antibody) could eliminate offending cross-reacting infectious agents such as poliovirus or toxins. He started giving injections of diluted venom to believers with a variety of illnesses, many of whom gave testimonials claiming improvement. When the serpentarium in South Miami closed around 1980, the source of the venom disappeared, but the myth continued. After having examined many dozens of MS patients who had received venom over a period of years, I concluded that there was no evidence that they had benefited from their experience. This was so, even though published research has revealed antiviral activity in the natural snake venom.

Bee Venom

Folk remedies are often applied with great conviction and ceremony. One of these, originating in the jungles of South America, is the practice of applying bee stings for **arthritis**. Several years ago a scientific study was carried out that initially seemed to confirm some benefit from the practice. Subsequently, purification of the venom was performed in an attempt to find a marketable product. This led to the finding of a single protein in the bee venom that was thought to be the active ingredient. Unfortunately, this purified protein failed to relieve arthritis, and scientific research was halted.

Claims that bee stings offer a therapeutic benefit for MS have no scientific basis. No pharmaceutical company is likely to pursue this issue. There is real potential harm to MS patients who are immunosuppressed from certain treatments such as steroids, azathioprine (Imuran), or methotrexate. There are **tetanus** spores in bee venom, and in immunosuppressed patients, germination of these spores can lead to tetanus, which is potentially fatal. The only notable effects in MS patients that I have witnessed have been allergic reactions complicated by serious deterioration, ending in death in a small number of MS patients. We have never used nor recommended bee venom as a treatment for MS.

A word of warning: Any lay person can walk into health food store and be met with multiple unfounded claims for products that can be obtained without prescription. *Buyer Beware!*

70. Is there anything I can do about my overwhelming fatigue?

In contrast to the lack of effective remedies in health food stores, we currently have effective treatments for fatigue. Amantadine is a drug that was approved more

Arthritis

A term commonly used to describe joint disease causing pain. It should, however, be reserved for inflammatory disease of joints, as rheumatoid arthritis.

Treatment

Tetanus

A potentially fatal illness produced by infection with the bacterium Clostridium tentani , most often complicating wound contamination. It is characterized by rapidly increasing stiffness and may lead to seizures and death.

than 35 years ago to prevent and subsequently treat influenza. It has also been proven to be of benefit in reducing fatigue in MS. Drugs such as amphetamine and Ritalin have been used, but none is as safe and well tolerated as amantadine. Moreover, habituation to Ritalin and amphetamine occurs quickly. More recently, modafinil (Provigil), which was approved for management of narcolepsy, has been prescribed in MS with limited effectiveness. Tolerance seems to develop quickly in some patients, and higher doses are often not well tolerated. Some patients do experience a sustained improvement. Importantly, the drug is relatively expensive.

Karen's comment:

My family and I refer to fatigue as "fat-goo" after a kind, but inexperienced, nurse trainee who was unfamiliar with the word pronounced it the way it feels—like I'm trying to go through fat and goo to function. I am unable to will myself to do something that I feel I should otherwise be able to do. What I find most difficult about fatigue is managing it psychologically. I get tired of being tired. Sometimes I feel as if I should try harder to get "through the goo," but usually when I try this I end up falling, dropping something, and overloading cognitively. Then I have more to do when I am functioning again.

Fatigue is also hard on others psychologically. It is an invisible symptom—part of the "but you look so good" phenomenon. This is when well-meaning people will look at me and say to themselves or to me, "I would never know you had an illness; you look so good." They have no idea how hard it is to function and perform everyday tasks such as brushing my teeth, getting dressed, and sitting up in a chair—much less walking.

I treat my fatigue with Amantadine, caffeine (preferably Cuban colada), and sugar in a form that I can carry with me and take in small portions, such as M&Ms and jelly beans. These "medicines" do not always get me through, but they help. The other remedy for fatigue is getting help—volunteer and paid. For me, one of the biggest parts of acceptance of MS has been asking for help. I am a very private (at least before contributing to this book) and independent person. The balance and choice are between help and independence, need and want, staying in the world and isolation, and safety and danger.

I have certain activities that I prefer to do alone but can no longer do safely. Thus, I forgo the activity, modify it, or have a "spotter" at the ready. Take, for example, showering; it is not safe for me to shower alone; however, it is an activity that I need to do, and my husband often travels. Thus, in lieu of dirt, when I shower, I have someone with me. I call someone when I get in and when I get out, or I have someone on the speakerphone. My sister, who lives nearby, is a CPA; thus, I know if I want to shower during tax season, she is at her desk at all hours. One time I called her back at the end of my shower, and I said, "I am out. I am clean. I am wet, and I am naked." After a pause, I heard discreet coughing in the background, and she said, "And you are also on the speakerphone in our conference room." I have not visited her at work since.

For activities I should not do alone I have wonderful friends: one who regularly gets up at 5 AM and another with whom I bake, bike, and play bridge. My family is very willing to keep me company doing activities that they had not done previously. One sister started ballet in her 40s, and my father began yoga in his 70s. Before taking me to the MRI the day I was diagnosed, my father had never accompanied me to a doctor, much less been part of the visit. Now he goes with me, and sometimes I even allow him to ask questions!

During a long flare-up, we decided to hire an aide for one day a week. It was hard to take this step, but those around us expressed relief and voiced surprise that I had not done this earlier. I was blessed to find a nurse who is flexible and understands my situation. During bad days she gets me up, does range of motion exercises, makes breakfast, and gets my medicine. On the good days, we have fresh-picked strawberries, deliver food to shut-ins, and run errands. When I told my family about hiring her, they were at first very defensive and felt that they should do these things with and for me. Now that time has passed we all have experienced the benefit she gives us. I am more independent and physically safer. My family members have one day a week that they are not on-call and can relax knowing that I am with a great professional. It helps, and we are all less fatigued.

71. What can I do about getting rid of this stiffness in my legs? What is the best treatment for spasticity?

A feeling of stiffness often is symptomatic of spasticity, although it may occur for other reasons. If you have cramps in your calves, especially at night, the problem is probably spasticity, for which there are a number of different therapies. If, however, a feeling of stiffness is due to impaired sensation in the legs, these treatments will not help.

Runners and other athletes use stretching of muscles to relieve muscle cramps. Not surprisingly, the first proven approach to the treatment of spasticity consisted of stretching the affected muscles. In the last 3 decades, several drugs have been proven to be helpful, including Valium (diazepam), Lioresal (baclofen), and Zanaflex (tizanidine). A single 5-mg dose of Valium at night is often sufficient for milder forms of spasticity. It has the advantage of being very long acting, and thus, if the spasticity is not severe, a single dose at nighttime may be sufficient for the entire day.

Baclofen (Lioresal) can be effective, but many patients do not get an effect that is proportional to the dose (that is, they have a poor dose response). Actually, Valium and baclofen have the same biochemical effect that reduces spasticity. Usually there is no need to give additional daytime doses of Valium. If 5- to 10-mg doses of Valium cause excessive daytime sedation or if these doses are insufficient to control stiffness or muscle cramps, the use of baclofen or tizanidine may be necessary. Tizanidine (Zanaflex) is a newer drug that has the advantage of not trading spasticity for weakness. However, it may produce drowsiness and intolerable dryness of the mouth. Baclofen and tizanidine can be used together for additional benefit. Tizanidine is not usually prescribed with Valium because of excessive sedation. Another drug, dantrolene hydrochloride (Dantrium), is used infrequently because of its potential liver toxicity. Although they are commonly used, all of these drugs should be prescribed and monitored by a neurologist who can assess their effectiveness.

Karen's comment:

Spasticity for me has ranged from slight stiffness to extreme stiffness that makes me look like a mechanical doll. In between the extremes is tightness. If I get into the wrong position, I require another person to "untangle me." Sometimes there is a lot of pain, and other times it is painless.

My first experience with Baclofen left me so weak from one pill that I could barely sit up or function for 3 days; thus, I have not retried it. When I took Tegretol, I threw up from each dose and felt very unlike myself—almost altered and distanced from my own being. So I have not retried it either. When I took Neurontin, I immediately threw up despite the minor dose.

During a severe episode of spasticity, we were reluctant to try medication. I spent 3 days stiff and in extreme pain. In desperation, my husband carried me into the swimming pool that we are fortunate enough to have in our back yard. My muscles relaxed, and I fell asleep in his arms. My husband is very intelligent; however, he had not thought through what to do in this circumstance: 2 AM, holding a sleeping wife in a pool with no phone or book nearby. He lasted 3 hours and woke me with both of us resembling prunes! For the next few days, when I would start to stiffen up, I would get into the pool, and it would pass. After several nights of splashing, moans, and groans coming from our side of the fence, our neighbors finally got up the nerve to ask us what exactly we were doing in the middle of the night!

For more "normal" spasticity, I stretch at yoga class and ballet class. In addition, I have others stretch me: professionals help two times a week, and my family is now trained at leaning, kneading, and pushing the various parts of me that need it. I am not always able to do the yoga or ballet, and sometimes, the most that I can manage is getting into a leotard (not an easy feat at my age in any event) and getting to class. Yet the training and muscle memory and the feeling of doing things for my body that

*are not strictly therapeutic or medicinal are very empower-
ing. It stretches me to places I thought I would never go.*

72. Is it true that baclofen can be injected? How does that work?

Baclofen can be injected to reduce spasticity, but it is only available for injection into the spinal fluid using an implantable pump. Direct injection into the spinal fluid is used only as a test to evaluate the patient's response before implanting the pump. This device allows the baclofen to be delivered into the spinal fluid continuously. It is called **intrathecal** baclofen and is used only for patients with severe spasticity that cannot tolerate the side effects of or do not benefit from oral baclofen. The injectable drug differs in its composition, making it more effective. Ordinarily, intrathecal baclofen is not considered in ambulatory patients.

Intrathecal
inside the central
nervous system.

73. Is it true that Botox injections can be used to treat spasticity?

Yes. Botox can be used to relieve spasticity. However, only neurologists or specialists in physical rehabilitation who are familiar with the special problems that MS patients may encounter should use Botox. Generally, the use of this drug is reserved for patients who have severe spasticity with early contractures in a single muscle group, such as the **gastrocnemius**, and have failed management with stretching and the drugs previously discussed. Botox is not a panacea for the management of spasticity.

Gastrocnemius
the large calf muscle
that pulls and keeps
the foot down.

Treatment

74. Why do some patients with MS become unable to urinate when they have to urinate all day and night?

Detrusor muscle

muscle of the urinary bladder that forms the actual storage organ and is the largest part of the bladder.

Sphincter

a circular muscle that constricts a passage such as the urethra or anus.

Hyporeflexic bladder

decreased bladder reactivity as defined by urodynamic testing in a laboratory.

Incontinence

urinary incontinence; involuntary loss of bladder control.

Bladder function is complex. Emptying the bladder is the result of three parts of the bladder functioning in sequence. To empty the urine from the bladder effectively, the bladder wall (the **detrusor muscle**) has to contract. When the pressure in the bladder has reached the right level, and only then, the bladder neck will normally relax and then the internal **sphincter** will relax. If the external sphincter is relaxed, voiding will occur. Sometimes, early in the course of MS, the bladder may not contract normally, and the sphincter does not relax, thus preventing the bladder from emptying. This is a so-called **hyporeflexic bladder**. However, most bladders are hyperreflexic, and the patient feels the urge to urinate frequently, sometimes with a feeling of great urgency. At times, the bladder uncontrollably empties unexpectedly or prematurely, resulting in urinary **incontinence**.

Anticholinergic

drugs that block the effect of the hormone acetylcholine in the body and are called anticholinergic drugs.

Catheterization [Bladder]

removal of urine from the bladder by means of a urinary catheter (tube).

Treatment of bladder dysfunction is usually directed at relieving symptoms and reducing the risk of infection. Ditropan and other **anticholinergic** drugs are the mainstay of the treatment of urinary frequency and urgency. Unfortunately, these drugs tend to produce dryness of the mouth. Often, patients prefer to use the drugs only at night to reduce wakening and risk of incontinence. These drugs can be useful when patients with urinary frequency and urgency have to leave their homes. Urinary **catheterization** is sometimes necessary to achieve bladder emptying and can help prevent recurrent bladder infections and complicating kidney damage. If catheterization is recommended, it should be done regularly. All patients with such problems should be seen by a urologist who is familiar with MS.

TREATMENT OF MS ATTACKS

75. How are MS attacks treated? Why are there different drugs to treat attacks of MS?

MS is characterized by unpredictable attacks of neurologic symptoms that vary greatly in type and severity. After being diagnosed, all patients are familiar with at least one symptom. They are concerned about recovering from the difficulty as soon as possible. Generally, recovery follows all attacks whether treatment is given or not. The speed of recovery is the only predictable outcome that is affected by treatment.

If a patient cannot perform his or her responsibilities at home or at work, shortening these more severe attacks by using drugs would seem to be of paramount importance. However, adrenocorticotrophic hormone (ACTH), also called corticotrophin, is the only FDA-approved treatment for attacks (relapses) of MS. Nevertheless, currently, most neurologists prescribe either oral or high-dose intravenous steroids (methylprednisolone, Medrol) for exacerbations of MS. Some neurologists prescribe them chronically. There is no scientific basis for this practice. There are many potential side effects, however. Steroids do reduce fatigue in MS patients and often induce a sense of well-being. Their many side effects, however, do not justify their use for those reasons. The optic neuritis study did show accelerated recovery from attacks of optic neuritis after the use of IV methylprednisolone (Medrol). In con-

Progressive multifocal leukoencephalopathy (PML)

a serious infection of the brain caused by the JC papilloma virus.

Cataracts

any opacification (loss of transparency) of the lens or its capsule.

Osteoporosis

a disease characterized by low bone mass and structural deterioration of bone tissue, leading to bone fragility and an increased risk of fractures of the hip, spine, and wrist.

Necrosis

tissue death; a state of irreversible tissue damage.

trast, oral steroids had no effect except to double the risk of relapse of optic neuritis as compared with IV Medrol. There often is a rapid response to either drug in patients with acute, severe relapses, but there are no good studies of either IV compared with any dose of oral steroids to evaluate this in MS. The side effects of steroids include an increased risk of infection, including viral, bacterial, yeast, fungal, and parasitic types. This includes **progressive multifocal leukoencephalopathy (PML)**, which has been recently reported in two study patients treated with Avonex and Tysabri. Other complications include psychiatric problems, **cataracts, osteoporosis**, and ischemic **necrosis** of hips and other joints (as well as others).

Karen's comment:

To steroid or not to steroid? Dr. Sheremata is in the minority on this issue. However, I have followed his advice not to take the customary steroids and instead consider rest and ACTH. Despite the side effects of steroids and the factual knowledge that we have about them, it has been hard not to take them when I have a flare-up.

When I have a flare-up, I will call or e-mail Dr. Sheremata and ask him to remind us again about his view. The desire on my part and those around me is to do something to alleviate the flare-up. The fear, the lack of control, the symptoms themselves, and the uncertainty all make it difficult to take the rest approach and not to take the steroid approach. However, I have followed the rest regimen, and I believe that I have recovered faster and stronger than if I had gone the steroid route. Furthermore, I do not have to recover from the steroids. Nonetheless, if and when I have my next flare-up, I imagine I will still re-ask the question.

Perhaps this book should be titled 100 Times the Same Questions About MS Are Asked!

76. What is ACTH?

ACTH (or corticotrophin) is a hormone that is made in the brain and is stored in the **pituitary gland**, which is situated at the base of the brain. This hormone is normally released in miniscule amounts during the early hours of the morning to stimulate the **adrenal glands'** production of steroid hormones. **Cortisol,** the active form of **cortisone**, is one product of ACTH stimulation. Dr. Leo Alexander began using ACTH a half-century ago at Harvard Medical School. He showed in a series of studies that it speeded recovery from MS attacks. Later, a national study, published in 1970, proved that it did indeed significantly speed the recovery for patients with acute exacerbations of MS.

ACTHAR gel, the commercial product, was withdrawn from the market when Parke Davis stopped manufacturing many drugs a number of years ago. However, as a result of the efforts of The National Organization for Rare Diseases (NORD) and the recognition of the value of ACTH, ACTHAR gel is again available. The intravenous form of ACTHAR is no longer available, and the synthetic form for intravenous use is in extremely short supply.

A quarter century of research has shown that ACTH also has neuroprotective properties, although clinical neurologists are rarely aware of this fact. In recent scientific studies of experimental optic neuritis at MIT in Boston, it has been shown that high-dose IV steroids

Treatment

Pituitary gland

an endocrine gland about the size of a pea at the base of the brain. The pituitary gland secretes hormones regulating a wide variety of bodily activities.

Adrenal glands

glands secrete steroid hormones that are important in the body's response to stress.

Cortisol

the primary steroid hormone produced by the adrenal gland. It is the biologically active soluble form of cortisone.

Cortisone

the stored form of cortisol produced by the adrenal cortex.

actually induce the death of brain nerve cells, the opposite effect of ACTH.

77. Why aren't drugs used together to get a better effect?

ACTH and IV steroids aren't ordinarily used together. However, high-dose IV steroids (in 1-gram daily doses) could be used for a 3- to 5-day period in patients who have especially severe attacks to reduce swelling in the optic nerve or spinal cord, with ACTH added to maintain adrenal function (since steroids suppress the adrenal glands) and thereby obtain the benefit of the other actions of ACTH. This would also provide the neuroprotective effect of ACTH.

Although you may ask why not continue the high-dose IV steroids, it is important to realize that high-dose steroids damage myosin, which is the main protein in muscle that is responsible for muscle contraction. Prolonged use of intravenous steroids may result in serious muscle damage, sometimes referred to as "intensive care unit paralysis." This is yet another reason why it is unwise to continue high-dose steroids for longer periods.

78. How do these drugs compare?

There is a lack of studies that address this issue of treatment comparisons. The optic neuritis study was the first attempt to compare oral versus IV steroids and placebo. This study failed to show any benefit from oral steroids. A small study in England revealed similar outcomes for IV steroids and ACTH; however, the numbers of patients were very small, and the study consequently suffered from problems in statistical analysis of the results (a Type II error). Essentially, a Type II error occurs when you compare two treatments in a study and there aren't a sufficient number of patients on each of the treatments. As a result, the benefits may *seem* not to be different, but the results are not valid. There are a number of other small studies from which valid conclusions are not possible. Valid studies have to be large and as a result are very expensive to conduct.

79. Why should I take drugs that have side effects?

This is an excellent question. Although patients recover from attacks of MS with or without drug treatment, recovery is hastened with ACTH treatment.

In the 1970 national study, MS patients in relapse were all placed at rest in hospitals. In this relatively small study, despite being in hospitalized and benefiting from rest, actively treated patients receiving ACTH were significantly better after 1, 2, and 3 weeks of ACTH treatment compared with those receiving placebo injections. Although the patients had less disability at 4 weeks (1 week after termination of treatment) as compared with placebo recipients, the difference was not statistically significant. Other studies probably should have been done to answer questions of dose as well as those related to dose forms, but they weren't. Despite their importance, it is unlikely that any such studies will be carried out on a significant scale anytime in the future.

It should be appreciated that physical rest, without the addition of drugs, is in itself beneficial and will result in faster recovery from attacks of MS. Recovery will eventually prevail to the extent that recovery will occur in any given attack. There is no evidence that treatment of MS attacks with any available treatment results in superior long-term results. In general, if an attack is minor, treatment does not provide any advantage and is better avoided. For example, if a person has decreased vision to 20/40 or even 20/60 in one eye, vision will return without treatment, often quite quickly. Apart from the cost, high-dose steroids certainly have potential side effects and would be best avoided in such an attack. However, based on our experience, in those rare patients who suffer a complete loss of vision in one or both eyes, high-dose steroids result in the recovery of usable vision in a greater proportion of patients.

80. What are the side effects of the drugs that are used for treatment of MS attacks? Are cataracts a result of steroid use? Is osteoporosis a complication of MS?

Side effects of steroids are common whether they are administered by mouth or IV. There are several categories of side effects: alteration of mood, formation of cataracts, increased risk of infection, impaired wound healing, loss of calcium from bone, ischemic necrosis of bone, and muscle damage, to mention only the more commonly recognized problems.

Cataracts: Cataracts are a well-known complication of steroid use. The risk of cataracts is related to the total dose of steroid used but varies greatly from person to person. The type of cataract is unique to the use of steroids and is easily recognized by **ophthalmologists**. As with other cataracts, extraction with lens replacement is the only real treatment. There seems to be little or no risk associated with ACTH use in MS.

Ophthalmologists
Physicians specialized in the diagnosis and treatment of diseases of the eye.

Treatment

Weight gain and altered body habitus: Steroids and ACTH result in an increased appetite. Their use can result in tremendous weight gain, even as high as 70 pounds in a few days. There is also a redistribution of body fat that women in particular do not like. Fat is deposited over the face and upper part of the chest and neck, abdomen, and buttocks. As easy as it is to gain the weight, it is difficult to take it off. When caloric intake is managed (restricted), the deposition of fat over the upper back, abdomen, and buttocks is minimized, but not eliminated. The alteration of body image may be traumatic, particularly to women. Acne often accompanies the use of steroids and ACTH. It can be easily managed with use of low doses of tetracycline antibiotics.

Infection: Infections complicating the use of steroids include an increased risk of infection of all types, including viral, bacterial, fungal, and parasitic disease. Although viral infections are usually mentioned as a risk with steroid administration, including a risk of progressive multifocal leukoencephalopathy (PML), these infections are relatively uncommon. **Shingles** (herpes zoster) and flares of **genital herpes** are probably the most common viral infections seen.

Shingles
skin infection caused by the herpes zoster virus.

Genital herpes
a contagious viral infection primarily affecting the genitals of men and women caused by the herpes simplex-2 virus (HSV-2).

Cystitis

inflammation of the bladder associated with symptoms of urinary frequency and urgency.

Pyelonephritis

an acute infection of the kidney associated with fever, contrasting with cystitis (a bladder infection) where fever does not occur.

Thrush

throat infection by the yeast Candida albicans. It commonly complicates treatment with antibiotics and steroids.

Yeast vaginitis

a common infection due to the yeast Candida albicans.

Systemic infections

as opposed to a localized infection, a system infection is any infection that causes generalized symptoms.

Toxoplasmosis

infestation of the human body by the one celled animal Toxoplasma gondii.

Pneumocystis

a one cell organism that causes rapidly fatal lung infestations in AIDS patients.

Compared with viral infections, bacterial infections are a more practical problem. The most commonly encountered bacterial infections complicating the use of steroids include flare-ups of bladder and kidney infections (**cystitis** and **pyelonephritis**). Less commonly, skin wounds, pneumonias, and rarer infections can be problematic.

Although yeast infestation of throat (**thrush)** and **yeast vaginitis** are relatively common problems with steroid treatment, they are usually generally easy to manage. **Systemic infections** are rare, but these can occasionally be very serious. Fungal infections are unusual except accompanying chronic steroid use.

Parasitic infections such as **toxoplasmosis** and **pneumocystis**, which complicate HIV infection, are not common, but they may complicate chronic steroid use, particularly if the steroids are used in combination with drugs such as Imuran and methotrexate.

Wound healing: Surgical and other wounds heal more slowly in patients on steroids and are more likely to become infected. For those with bed sores, steroids are particularly problematic. Management of these patients should avoid even short-term steroids.

Bone damage: The use of steroids results in the loss of calcium from bones that underlies the development of osteopenia and osteoporosis. Subsequently, this may lead to the collapse of vertebrae and an increased risk of fracture of the long bones. Even more serious is the increased likelihood of ischemic (aseptic) necrosis of the hips and other joints. When diagnosed early, treatment can reverse or limit permanent damage. Conversely, advanced joint damage leaves only joint replacement as an option. Physicians and patients have to be aware of such potential complications. Difficulty in walking or pain in the knee may actually signify or indicate damage to a hip rather than a knee. In my long experience, I have never seen this complication in ACTH-treated patients.

Muscle damage: Steroid therapy by any route, but especially with high-dose IV administration, weakens muscles. High-dose IV therapy carries with it the risk of severe muscle weakness, which fortunately, is usually reversible. This complication is not seen with ACTH.

81. Why do I go crazy with steroids?

In most patients, there is an initial feeling of well-being induced by steroids, particularly at lower doses. However, mood elevation often is replaced by irritability with continued administration, particularly at higher doses. Psychotic behavior may follow simple mood elevation. Frank **manic psychosis** occurs in a small proportion of patients treated with steroids by any route of administration. Mood elevation can be managed using lithium carbonate and diazepam. Although it is the more common response, other patients may become depressed. ACTH may also occasionally be associated with these mood changes.

Manic psychosis
a state of elevated mood and psychosis.

82. How do the side effects compare?

The side effects of ACTH are generally similar to those of steroids taken orally or by IV administration, but are less severe. All of the side effects seen with steroids, including psychosis but excluding muscle weakness and bone injury, may occur with ACTH. Certain hormones induced by ACTH and produced by the adrenal glands, the "keto-steroids" (like testosterone), have an anabolic (protein building) effect. In other words, as in athletes, anabolic steroids that are induced by ACTH treatment are capable of making muscles somewhat stronger. In contrast, the net effect of steroids is catabolic (protein destroying).

Karen's comment:

When I was first diagnosed with MS, my doctor at the time prescribed steroids, specifically oral prednisone, intravenous steroid methylprednisolone, and then more oral prednisone. As a result, I was simultaneously dealing with the diagnosis, my body going through things it had never done before (such as vision loss, MRI, and spinal tap), emotionally managing the logistics of a nurse for the IV steroids, processing the mounds of insurance forms, and coping with the side effects of the steroids.

Fortunately, I have low blood pressure, am not overweight, and manage my diet well, so I missed many of the side effects—however, not all. I got the telltale "Cabbage Patch Doll" face such that my eyeglasses would barely squeeze on. For several months, I was "hyper" and unable to sleep from midnight to 4 AM. I would alphabetically arrange our 1,000 books. Other odd things happened, such as when the hair on my arms fell out.

Coming off the steroids was hard as well. My body was addicted. One day I yelled at my husband for eating a potato chip too loudly when he was three rooms away. On another day, I felt a loss of adrenaline and ate an entire box of Dots candy I grabbed from the shelf of our grocery store. All told, from first dose to last weaning pill, I had 6 months of steroids—2 months of intended benefit and 4 months for withdrawal. Almost 10 years later I still have residual effects from that one event with steroids: I have some change in my body shape that is referred to as trunk effect, osteoporosis, and pre-cataract fibers in my eyes.

83. I don't want steroids. Are other treatments available for MS attacks?

Traditionally, the management of MS centered on the use of extended periods of physical (and mental) rest, as it did for patients with tuberculosis or **rheumatoid arthritis**. Today, relapse management in MS seems to revolve around the use of steroids. ACTH was approved for the treatment of attacks of MS by the FDA in 1978 and remains the only drug approved for treatment of MS attacks. The IV form of ACTH is in very short supply, but the intramuscular form (ACTHAR Gel) is again in production and can be obtained with a prescription.

Rheumatoid arthritis

a common inflammatory joint disease caused by an autoimmune response.

84. Why are IV steroids given for attacks of MS?

More than 30 years ago, after performing **myelograms** to rule out tumors, we found that the spinal cord was swollen during severe attacks of MS, causing paralysis. When CT scans of the brain and orbits became available to study patients with severe attacks of optic neuritis, we also found the optic nerves to be markedly swollen. We reasoned that with high doses of steroids we should be able to reduce the swelling in the spinal cord and optic nerve to prevent further damage from the lack of circulation in the affected areas of the ner-

Myelogram

x-ray studies of the spinal cord and spinal canal performed by the injection of contrast media. CT and MRI studies have replaced this procedure.

vous system. High-dose steroids did seem to work, often more quickly than with ACTH. However, many more side effects were found in patients with the use of high-dose steroids than with ACTH, which somewhat dissuaded us from using this form of treatment. Many neurologists favor the use of steroids as being convenient, disregarding the lack of adequate controlled trials in MS.

The optic neuritis trial of IV methylprednisolone (Medrol) appeared to validate the use of a high dose (1 gram per day) as effective in speeding recovery. Oral steroids, in contrast, did not accelerate recovery; their use resulted in a relapse rate that was twice as high in that trial. Although many neurologists have rationalized their prescription of oral steroids because of fatigue reduction and often restoration of a sense of well-being, they ignore a potentially higher post treatment relapse rate. Oral steroids have not been demonstrated in any adequate trial to be useful treatment for optic neuritis or other MS relapses.

85. Are there treatments to prevent attacks and lessen risk of disability?

Successful clinical and MRI study results for four drugs resulted in FDA approval of their marketing for the treatment of relapsing MS. The first was interferon-beta-1b (Betaseron) in 1993, interferon-beta-1a (Avonex in 1996 and Rebif in 2002), and glatiramer acetate (Copaxone) in 1997. There is a marked reduction in new MRI lesions within the first month with the higher dose interferon product Betaseron and by inference with Rebif. However, none of these drugs reveals any reduction of relapse rates within 6 months of initiation of treatment. After 2 years of treatment, exacerbations are reduced by approximately 30% for each of these approved products. Although subcutaneous interferon-beta-1b (Betaseron) and interferon-beta-1a (Rebif) have similar salutary reductions in exacerbations at 1 year, this is not seen in this time frame with Avonex or with Copaxone. The higher dose interferons have more side effects associated with them with their initial use. Both high-dose forms of interferon-beta are associated with injection site reactions as well as significant "flu-like" reactions, principally consisting of fever, headache, and diffuse aches and pains. Local skin reactions may be prominent. These side effects become less severe and may disappear within a few weeks of initiating therapy. Glatiramer acetate, similarly, is associated with injection site reactions about half as frequently (about 40%) and an anxiety-like syndrome with chest tightness in a smaller proportion of patients. A flu-like syndrome is relatively uncommon in glatiramer-treated patients.

Natalizumab (Tysabri) in MS

The clinical outcomes in the Phase III trials of natalizumab (Tysabri) greatly surpassed those of the products currently available. Natalizumab reduced the risk of sustained disability at 2 years by 42%. In MRI studies, a similar early reduction in gadolinium-enhancing lesions was seen with high-dose interferon-beta as with natalizumab.

The AFFIRM (natalizumab safety and efficacy in relapsing-remitting MS) study was a 2-year, multicenter, randomized, placebo-controlled investigation of a fixed intravenous 300-mg dose of natalizumab every 4 weeks. Of the total enrollment of 942 patients, 627 patients received active treatment. On the basis of the primary outcome for the first year, a 66% reduction of relapses and a favorable safety and tolerance profile for the drug led to its approval for the prevention of relapses in November 2004. The primary outcome measure for the completed 2-year study was the impact of treatment on the prevention of sustained disability (defined as a 3-month increase in disability by one point on the EDSS). The reduction of relapses was sustained through the second year, with a 42% reduction in sustained disability. Using the same criteria used in the Avonex trial (sustained disability by one point on the EDSS for 6 months), a 56% reduction was reported.

The SENTINEL (safety and efficacy of natalizumab in combination with Avonex [interferon-beta-1a]) study was a second ongoing 2-year randomized multi-center, placebo-controlled, double-blind study of 1,171 relapsing-remitting MS patients. The same dose of natalizumab (300 mg IV every 4 weeks) was used. In this trial, patients who had been treated with Avonex (interferon beta-1a) but who had experienced one or more relapses while on treatment were randomized to receive natalizumab or placebo on a 1:1 basis. Avonex was continued throughout the study for both groups. The Avonex group consisted of 582 patients, and the combined treatment group had 589 patients. The outcome measures for this second 2-year study were the same as those for the AFFIRM study. Natalizumab reduced the frequency of relapse by 54% versus placebo.

Despite the marked salutary effect on relapses, the fact that the full impact of the drug on relapses was realized by 6 weeks of treatment and the accompanying reduction of sustained disability, the drug has been withdrawn from the market. The withdrawal was necessary because, unfortunately, 2 of the 589 patients who had received Avonex and Tysabri (one for 23 and the other for 37 months) developed PML, a fatal opportunistic viral disease of the brain. In addition, a patient with Crohn's disease who had received multiple drug therapies also developed this disease. Of the approximately 3,000 patients with MS, Crohn's disease, or rheumatoid arthritis, the only patients who developed PML were those two MS patients on combined Tysabri and Avonex therapy and the Crohn's disease patient who had received multiple immunosuppressants as well as Tysabri. The drug has been withdrawn from the market pending a full review of the relevant facts.

Karen's comment:

I took Tysabri in 1997 and in 2004. In October 1997, I was feeling great. My MS was seemingly nonexistent. I was in New Jersey enjoying the fall leaves, biking, and picking raspberries; I even thought about trying to teach in the spring term. I did not realize that I was pregnant and soon to miscarry. After the miscarriage, we called Dr. Sheremata, who asked when I was next going to be in Miami. I told him in a week, for my father's 65th birthday. He warned us that it was likely that I would have a flare-up. As I enjoyed a long weekend in Florida, I felt a bit smug and a lot relieved that I had not had a flare-up and almost canceled my appointment with Dr. Sheremata for that Tuesday. Monday night I was tired but still okay. By Tuesday morning I could not see out of my right eye, and neither of my legs worked very well. My father and I went to see Dr. Sheremata; we discussed ACTH, and Dr.

Sheremata mentioned a drug trial. The Phase 2 study was designed for patients who were within 48 hours of the beginning of a flare-up, and I was certainly in that group. I had to agree to be studied for 3 months at regular intervals, including MRIs, physical exams, and blood work. Insult to injury—I had to take a pregnancy test to make sure that I was not pregnant. The Informed Consent Agreement was standard, and what I had seen as sensible as a practicing lawyer seemed ridiculous as a patient in the midst of a flare-up—ill and with poor vision, how informed could I be about an experiment for something only a few humans had tried? The prior trial for a different MS drug had been halted when patients had what the FDA termed "strong negative events" (i.e., heart attacks). I called my husband in New Jersey, who just as when I was first diagnosed with MS was worried and had difficulty imagining how I could be so ill because 2 days ago when he had seen me I was fine. I felt a bit like the castaways on Gilligan's Island. I had left for a 3-day weekend to be gone for 3 months as a guinea pig. How did we decide to do the trial? We prayed.

The next day another patient and I had infusions of drug or placebo. Over many hours Dr. Sheremata observed us. My father nervously ate the sandwiches, as the other patient and I were too tense to eat, and my husband called regularly. As we left the hospital and went over the bridge to the island where we live, I thought about what I had done; I wondered if my hair had turned purple. I wondered what was happening in my body. I could not undo it. The next day I felt great. The independent doctor who was doing the physical exams said I either got drug or had great prayer and placebo. During my exam before I had the IV, he had told me that I needed a foot brace and a walker. Now I was biking 10 miles. It turned out that I received *the drug and not placebo, and as always, I had great prayer.*

86. Is there treatment that stops MS?

As noted previously here, several treatments have now been proven in a series of trials to reduce the risk of relapses in MS. The newest drug, Tysabri, has the greatest benefit in this regard, with a 66% reduction in relapses. Although in their respective trials most of the drugs have been shown to decrease the risk of progression, it is not correct to say that they are capable of stopping MS. The benefits of Betaseron, Avonex, Rebif, and Tysabri appear somewhat similar in this regard. Some MS patients have milder illness than others, and aggressive management, with consequent more prominent side effects, may not be indicated. However, as outlined previously here, Tysabri has just recently been withdrawn from the market by Biogen-Idec and Elan pending review of unexpected complications.

There is evidence that Novantrone, the most aggressive treatment approved, stabilizes the majority of progressive, or worsening, MS patients. Although it may be tempting to use this more aggressive treatment in patients with relapsing-remitting MS, as is being done in Europe, important side effects from this drug must be considered. Although all forms of treatment for MS (and virtually all medical conditions) have side effects, the specific issues associated with Novantrone, such as the risk of leukemia (rare) and cardiac complications, cannot be ignored.

Karen's comment:

Tysabri comes close to stopping my MS. As with any experimental drug, there are many obstacles and checkpoints before it gets to market, if at all. Tysabri seems to have had one of the longer and more roller coaster-like routes to market and beyond. On November 23, 2004, 7 years after my drug trial infusion, the FDA approved Tysabri.

During the 7 years I went through as many changes as the corporations that owned the drug and then some. I had over 15 flare-ups, tried (without benefit) an interferon, volunteered for several drug trials that did not materialize, spent over a year at a 5.5 disability level, lost function in several areas, and considered chemotherapy. The day after FDA approval, our local pharmacist ordered a vial of Tysabri for me. On December 21, 2004, I took it to the doctor in our "playmate cooler" and had an infusion, one of the first in the world.

After the first infusion, I slept for 3 days and woke up stronger and stayed stronger than I had been for many years. There were no negative side effects. I felt like I was going to get a chance to get better. I had been having flare-ups every few months and felt like Sisyphus—each time I would get even a foothold, I would get rolled back down the mountain of MS. Two infusions later, the drug was withdrawn from the market and now, again, we wait.

87. Would starting the ABC drugs prevent progression of MS? Will it really make a difference?

Yes! The so-called ABC drugs (Avonex, Betaseron, and Copaxone) have been proven to reduce the risk of attacks in relapsing forms of MS. The original interferon-beta-1b (Betaseron) studies reported in 1993 (leading to approval later that year) were not designed to show a reduction in the risk of disability. The subsequent interferon-beta-1a (Avonex and Rebif) studies were designed to detect the impact of treatment on preventing "sustained" disability, as well as the impact on relapse rates. More recently, the benefit of Betaseron in reducing the risk of progression in secondary progressive disease was established. This was a more difficult task and was not found in studies of other interferon-beta products. Interestingly, this reduction in the risk of progression in the Betaseron studies was only evident in patients who continued to relapse as well as exhibit progression of their illness.

Using drugs does make a difference in MS. Studies have proven that the interferon-beta products (Avonex, Betaseron, and Rebif) approved for the use in MS have a benefit not only in reducing the risk of attacks but also the risk of "sustained" disability (progression), although it is not realized in everybody taking these drugs.

The pivotal studies of Copaxone did not show an impact on prevention of disability. A 6-year longitudinal follow-up study of a portion of the original study participants has been interpreted to show an impressive prevention of disability in about two thirds of those followed. There is no test than can predict therapeutic success; however, repeated examinations by experienced neurologists and MRI scans can provide information about how an individual patient is responding to treatment. Generally, apart from examinations and MRI scans, if you feel well, you probably are okay.

88. How do these drugs compare?

To date, there have only been two comparative drug studies in MS, and only one of these, the EVIDENCE trial, had good quality (blinded) data collection. This comparison of interferon-beta-1a at 30 mcg intramuscularly (IM) weekly (Avonex) to 44 mcg three times weekly (Rebif) was a single blind design study. The study did show superior results at 6, 12, and 16 months in favor of the higher dose (Rebif). Interestingly, the data from the earlier pivotal studies of both drugs showed similar outcomes in patients completing 2 years, as the investigators reported. It would appear that in the short term, at least, early institution of high-dose (44 mcg three times weekly) interferon-beta-1a (Rebif) is more efficacious than low dose (30 micrograms once weekly) (Avonex).

89. How do (approved) drugs used in MS prevent attacks?

Interferon-alpha and then interferon-beta-1b were first used in MS studies because of their known antiviral properties. At the present time, however, there is no accepted evidence that acute or chronic viral infection itself has any role in the causation of MS attacks or progression. There have been numerous studies of what the interferons do in the human body and specifically how they affect mechanisms of tissue damage in MS. A number of effects that both interferons possess should have a favorable effect in MS.

Among other properties, interferons decrease the activation (turning on) of lymphocytes and macrophages in a number of different ways. Another effect is to decrease the ability of activated cells to stick to the inside of the blood vessels of the brain and spinal cord via adhesion molecules. The interferons also interfere with cells already stuck to the inside of the blood vessels and their ability to initiate the series of events that allow the cells to eat a hole through the blood vessel's wall. This is accomplished through a number of different mechanisms, including the inhibition of **metalloproteases (MMPs)**. It is generally accepted that these several mechanisms are important in the benefits of Betaseron, Avonex, and Rebif in MS.

Glatiramer acetate (Copaxone), although not an interferon, appears to behave as theorized. As designed, it seems to function as a decoy for the immune system. It prevents myelin-like proteins from activating mechanisms causing additional myelin damage. Extrapolating from animal studies, there appear to be a number of beneficial effects on immune function when using Copaxone. There is recent evidence that Copaxone plays an important role in MS by switching off cytotoxic lymphocytes (CD8+ cells) and turning on immunosuppressive activity.

Metalloproteases (MMPs)

members of a group of secreted neutral proteases that degrade the collagens of the extracellular matrix. Members of this group are important in maintaining and breaching the integrity of the blood-brain barrier.

90. Why aren't drugs used together to get a better effect?

In a form of shorthand that immunologists use, helper T-cell immune function is referred to as "CD4 Th1 function," and suppressor inducer T-cell (immunoregulatory) is referred to as a type of "CD4 Th2 function." The net result of both the interferons and glatimer acetate is to "shift immune function away from Th1 activity toward Th2 function." It would seem that the drugs used in combination might be more effective in altering immune function to increase CD4 Th2 function. Therefore, there may be additional benefit from the combination of these forms of treatment. A new pivotal study, the CombiRx study, designed to explore the potential benefit of interferon-beta-1a (Avonex) versus glatiramer acetate (Copaxone) versus the combination of these drugs, is now being initiated.

91. What is Tysabri, and why was the drug withdrawn from the market?

Natalizumab (Tysabri) is a monoclonal antibody to an adhesion molecule (VLA-4) that was approved November 2004 on the basis of a marked (66%) reduction of MS exacerbations, a 91% reduction in MRI gadolinium-enhancing brain lesions, and a good safety and tolerance profile. This reduced exacerbation rate was sustained through the entire 2 years of the study. In addition, these effects were accompanied by an impressive 42% reduction in the risk of sustained progression of disability for the 2 years of the study. The reduction in the risk of attacks was achieved by selectively blocking one, and only one, Velcro-like molecule on lymphocytes preventing them from attaching to the inside of brain and spinal cord (cerebral) blood vessels. Extrapolating from animal studies, this action effectively prevented the cells from crossing the blood-brain barrier. The dramatically superior effectiveness of Tysabri in preventing attacks of MS, which was also seen after 2 years of therapy, confirmed the importance of blood lymphocytes and macrophages in their role in attacks of MS, and also proved that this step (attachment via a specific adhesion molecule VLA-4) is a central factor in attacks of MS.

The apparent synergism of Tysabri and Avonex in suppressing immune function sufficiently to allow PML to occur in two MS patients on combined therapy, but not in any patient receiving Tysabri monotherapy, is a demonstration of the potency of blocking the adhesion molecule (VLA-4). The outcome of combining Tysabri and Avonex is also a demonstration of the potential hazards of combining other apparently safe effective therapies with a more potent therapy. As a consequence of the findings, Biogen-Idec and Elan Pharmaceuticals have withdrawn Tysabri from the market. All of the facts surrounding the appearance of PML in Tysabri-treated patients have been presented to an independent panel. The panel's recommendations and FDA action will be the basis of the use of the drug in the future. It is safe to say that any use will not include combination therapy with interferon-beta of any type.

92. What are the side effects of the drugs that are used to prevent attacks? Why should I take drugs that have side effects? How do the side effects compare?

The approved drugs reduce the risk of exacerbations as well as the risk of disability and were FDA approved because of their safety as well as their effectiveness. However, most recipients of the drugs available for MS treatment (Betaseron, Avonex, Rebif, and Copaxone) do experience side effects. Flu-like symptoms occur in the majority of patients early in interferon-beta therapy regardless of which one is chosen. Generally, they are more prominent for higher dose interferon-beta (Betaseron and Rebif) and less for low dose interferon-beta (Avonex) and for Copaxone. The higher dose interferons, however, have a more rapid onset of benefit, as judged from MRI studies and the pivotal drug study results.

Local reactions to injections under the skin (subcutaneous injections) are less frequent for Copaxone, about half as common as compared with injections of interferon-beta (Betaseron and Rebif). Localized redness of the skin decreases over time but almost always persists to some degree in the majority. Most patients readily accept it as a nuisance. A few people will develop little dents in the skin in areas where the drug has been injected, similar to areas where insulin has been administered in diabetics. Others will develop hard nodules under the skin at the injection site. Some patients who are given Avonex or Rebif experience some stinging sensation with injections, which may be due to the acidity of the solution.

Copaxone, despite daily injections, is associated with fewer side effects than the interferon-beta products, but the full benefit is delayed, as it is with Avonex. Copaxone induces a local reaction in about 40% of the patients; half complain of some pain at the injection site. This again does not appear to be a major problem. A few patients develop prominent skin rashes. Approximately one quarter of patients experience a transient feeling of anxiety or shortness of breath, which is ordinarily a minor issue, but occasionally, it is more severe and longer lasting.

In summary, it can be fairly stated that the side effects from Betaseron and Rebif are initially more prominent but tend to subside sooner than in patients treated with Avonex. Generally, the side effects from Copaxone are less severe. For all of the products, there are considerable differences from one individual to another. The reason why certain patients tolerate one drug better than others remains unknown.

93. What is "the vaccine for MS?"

There seems to be a great deal of confusion in the minds of many MS patients and their families about a vaccine for MS. Some seem to think of any injectable drug as a vaccine, but this is not a correct concept. All of the medications currently approved by the FDA for chronic (long-term) use in MS are drugs but are not considered to be vaccines, although their use is to prevent periods of ill health. Interferon-beta-1b (Betaseron) and interferon-beta-1a (Avonex and Rebif) and glatiramer acetate (Copaxone) are injectable drugs but are not vaccines. In contrast, a vaccine, which is generally injected, stimulates the immune system, resulting in antibody formation or a direct effect of lymphocytes against proteins or cells that have specific proteins on their surface. Several vaccines against cells in the immune system have been used in research trials.

94. Is there going to be a vaccine for MS?

There is ongoing research into T-cell vaccines for MS. The original experiments in Europe attracted great interest. They involved injecting crude preparations of blood lymphocytes into patients in an attempt to elim-inate or reduce the number of "activated" lymphocytes in MS patients. Ongoing studies involve a more

Treatment

sophisticated selection of cells to be targeted for removal by immune action. They appear to be tolerable and effective to a degree. They do not result in a long-lasting benefit. Other stalled studies attempted to induce immune tolerance without provoking a direct attack on existing cells; only preliminary data on their safety have been published. No studies of this third generation type of vaccine are continuing.

Hypnotism

the use of suggestion; the field of study which encompasses, among other things, hypnotic trance; its induction, management, and application; and related subjects such as the phenomena of waking suggestion. Hypnotherapy is defined as the use of therapeutic techniques or principles in conjunction with hypnosis.

Biofeedback

a training technique that enables a patient to gain voluntary control over autonomic function.

95. What does alternative medicine have to offer?

There is no lack of "alternative" approaches to the holistic management of MS or for specific or individual problems. The vast majority of these "therapies" are of questionable value, whereas some are potentially dangerous. However, in the right hands, **hypnotism** and **biofeedback** may be very helpful approaches.

96. Is hypnotism helpful in MS?

The use of hypnotism is not to be taken lightly. Certainly, only trained professionals who are aware of MS and who are in communication with the patients' treating physicians should use hypnotism. There is no generally accepted use of this modality in MS. However, there may be a place for hypnotism in combination with psychotherapy.

97. Is biofeedback useful in MS?

In recent years, biofeedback has become commonly used in the management of pain in pain clinics. The use of biofeedback now appears to be generally well accepted. However, in past studies with Dr. Ronald Melzack at McGill University, surprisingly, we found that Workman's Compensation patients with back pain responded better to biofeedback than MS patients with back pain did. Biofeedback, however, may be helpful in some MS patients. More sophisticated approaches to biofeedback have recently evolved from spinal cord injury centers and other medical clinics.

98. Is there a cure for MS in the near future?

The old aphorism "nothing is impossible, but some things are just more difficult" is an appropriate response to this challenge. A cure for MS is not likely. Just as men and women recover from heart attacks and lead productive lives, patients can function well with a diagnosis of MS.

Although a half century ago rational treatment of MS seemed improbable, if not impossible, treatments proven to reduce the risk of attacks and disability have become a reality in the last 12 years. Consequently, we all eagerly await new developments in the field of MS treatment. Better experimental treatment designs and more effective drugs are anticipated. If a drug is to be used, it first must be shown to be safe. Then, and only then, is it permissible to investigate the effectiveness of the new drug in patients.

A report of the preliminary efficacy studies of natalizumab (Tysabri) appeared in the *New England Journal of Medicine* 2 years ago. The pivotal study, reported at the annual American Academy of Neurology meeting

Treatment

in Miami Beach in April 2005, provided evidence that this new drug was even more effective than it had appeared to be earlier and provided the basis for FDA approval. Despite the excitement regarding its earlier appearance of safety and efficacy, it has now been withdrawn from the market for safety reasons. When combined with Avonex, it appears to be excessively immunosuppressive and resulted in PML in two cases. This new drug with its unique mechanism of action may be too effective to allow combination therapy, at least with interferons. The facts of the matter will have to be elucidated to determine whether it can be reintroduced for the treatment of MS.

Karen's comment:

One of my nieces was in an advanced science program at the age of 7 years. The class assignment was to invent something new; hers was to fix "Multiple Skleroys." Although her spelling was not accurate, her sentiment is one shared by many. When I was first diagnosed in 1996, the pundits predicted a cure for MS in 5 years. Five years later the anticipated cure was within 10 years. Now it is said, "Perhaps within my lifetime."

Over the years, my thinking about cure has also evolved—not just about an ever-extending time line but also the meaning of cure. As a retired lawyer and non-retired bibliophile, the definition of a word is important to me. "Cure"—does it mean all people who get MS after a cure is found will be made disease-free; all people who have MS now will become disease-free or symptom-free; existing MS brain and nerve damage will be repaired; or no one will get MS?

Until a cure is found, whatever it means, I view my role as threefold: to give my support, financial and other, to those people and organizations working on a cure; to volunteer my body, alive and dead, to researchers working on a cure; and to keep myself physically, mentally, and spiritually as strong as possible to be ready for a cure and to be ready if a cure is not found in my lifetime. I have confidence in my niece.

99. What is the future?

Advances in the therapy of MS and autoimmune disease in general will certainly continue just as they have in other disorders. Although T-cell vaccination has some promise, results to date have been somewhat disappointing, but those trials are continuing. A dream treatment of eliminating immune reactions aimed at myelin, a theoretical possibility, when given early in the course of disease could result in permanent cessation of clinical activity. This third-generation type of T-cell vaccine would induce permanent immune tolerance to an offending antigen (protein) and could be a "one-shot cure." There are no current trials in progress, but this approach will certainly be revisited.

With the improved understanding of disease mechanisms and the dangers and limitation of selective adhesion molecule modulation, it is anticipated that in the future oral drugs may replace the use of IV medication (Tysabri). Preliminary efficacy (Phase II) trials of a product employed by Glaxo-Smith Kline have apparently achieved results resembling those of natalizumab. If these drugs achieve similar or equal effectiveness and are safe, they will gain rapid acceptance. Because trials have been stopped, they will not become a reality in the immediate future. Other approaches blocking IL-12, a hormone essential to the immune cascade, with monoclonal antibodies are currently being employed by two pharmaceutical companies. Hopefully, these studies will lead to the availability of alternative safe and effective mechanisms of **immunomodulation** in MS. Because of the need to compare effectiveness of treatment rather than to compare a given treatment with placebo, fewer drugs are likely to enter future trials. However, a number of newer approaches to management are entering trials now, and only time will tell if they truly represent safer and/or more effective treatments.

The surprising new findings in Crohn's disease of a new genetic mutation in 80% of a subset of patients that provides a "rational" explanation for the illness seemed unlikely just a year ago. This is now is a reality; however, no one really anticipates finding an "MS" gene. However, this new finding in Crohn's disease exemplifies now that good genetic and biological research can provide unanticipated new discoveries in medicine. Research is the key to the future in MS, as it is for all of the biological sciences and in medicine.

Karen's comment:

Unpredictable, unknowable, and uncertain are all charac-teristics of the future for a person with MS. As a person of reason, I think that these characteristics hold true for every-one, MSers and non-MSers alike. As a person of faith, I believe that there is also hope.

Immunomodulation

treatment aimed at changing immune responses to benefit a patient with autoimmune disease.

100. Where can I get more information about MS?

It is not possible to discuss all of the aspects of MS in one small volume. The Appendix contains organizations, websites, and publications that can be useful to MS patients and their families.

Treatment

Appendix

Organizations

The National Multiple Sclerosis Society (NMSS)
It is headquartered in New York, has local chapters in most communities.
They publish educational pamphlets and sponsor research. Their website,
http://www.nmss.org, is one of the few truly helpful websites available to
MS patients and their families as well as to neurologists and other physicians.

Multiple Sclerosis International Federation
Information about MS in English, Spanish, French, Italian, German, and
Russian is available. International Portal provides access to member MS
Societies around the world. Their website (http://www.msif.org) has a link
from the NMSS.

Multiple Sclerosis Association of America (MSAA)
Although a smaller organization, MSAA is another important resource.
Their address is as follows: 706 Haddonfield Road, Cherry Hill, NJ 08002.
Telephone: (800) Learn MS. Their website is http://www.msaa.com.

The National Organization for Rare Diseases
This organization supports important MS relevant issues. Their website is
http://www.rarediseases.org/.

The Montel Williams Foundation
This is a newer foundation that is getting a lot of attention. Their focus is on research. 331 West 57th Street, PMB #420, New York, NY 10019. Their telephone is: 212-830-0343; Fax: 212-262-4608. Their website is http://www.montelms.org/.

Multiple Sclerosis Foundation
A number of other regional foundations, such as the Multiple Sclerosis Foundation in Fort Lauderdale, exist and provide important additional support for MS-related activities. Their address is 6350 North Andrews Avenue, Ft. Lauderdale FL 33309-2130. Telephone (888) 573-6287; Fax (954) 772-0867. Their website is http://www.msfacts.org/.

The Pharmaceutical Industry
The pharmaceutical industry sponsors websites that can provide helpful guidance, especially for the products they provide. The companies are listed alphabetically:

Berlex (Betaseron)
http://www.mspathways.com

Biogen-Idec (Avonex)
http://www.avonex.com/msavProject/avonex.portal

Serono (Rebif)
http://www.mslifelines.com

Teva (Copaxone)
http://www.mswatch.com/Community/

Publications

Roy Swank: A Diet for Multiple Sclerosis (Doubleday Publishers)
This book is based on a lifetime of interest, experience, and study. It is a winner. Dr. Swank spent his life studying MS.

Glossary

"ABC": A commonly used unofficial reference to Avonex-Betaseron-Copaxone as approved drugs for MS treatment.

Acinetobacter: A bacterium that infects the upper respiratory tract and that has been hypothesized to be a causative factor in MS by some researchers in England.

Acne: A skin condition common in young people with increased secretion from oil glands in the skin, accompanied by formation of comedos (blackheads). These glands tend to become infected with organisms living in or on the skin making the skin raised and red.

ACTH: Adrenocorticotrophic hormone (now also called corticotrophin), the hormone made in the brain and stored in the pituitary gland at the base of the brain. It is the only FDA-approved treatment for shortening MS attacks.

Acute disseminated encephalomyelitis: An acute spontaneous, postinfectious, or postvacinial central nervous system disease. It is characterized by simultaneous appearance of nervous system symptoms due to inflammation in the white matter of the brain and or the spinal cord, resembling an attack of MS. Unlike MS it ordinarily does not relapse in adults but may occasionally do so in children. It can be very serious but more often is a relatively mild illness.

Adhesion molecules: Velcro-like proteins on the surface of white blood and other cells that allow them to stick to the lining of veins.

Adrenal glands: Glands of internal secretion situated above the kidneys sometimes referred to as supra-renal glands. The cells of the cortex (on the outside of the gland) secrete cortisone and other steroid hormones that are important in the body's response to stress. Adrenaline and noradrenalin are hormones also secreted by nerve cells in the center (medulla) of the gland.

Adrenaline: The principal hormone secreted by the adrenal medulla. This hormone is made from the amino acid tyrosine and is not a steroid. It makes the heart beat more forcefully and faster and raises the blood pressure. Adrenalin secretion is also part of the "fight or flight" response to stress.

Antibody: Proteins made by the immune system to defend against infectious agents. At times, antibody may be directed against our own tissues, resulting in autoimmune disease. Antibody is produced when B-cells are stimulated by antigen.

Anticholinergic: Drugs that block the effect of the hormone acetylcholine in the body and are called anticholinergic drugs. These drugs include atropine, scopolamine, Ditropan, etc. and are used to slow the heart rate down, dry secretions, and reduce the contractions of bowel and bladder. These drugs produce dryness of the mouth and constipation as common side effects.

Antigen: An antigen is any substance (bacterium, virus, or single molecule), usually a protein, but sometimes a sugar or fat that stimulates an immune reaction in the body. This immune reaction may result in the production of antibody or a cellular immune reaction.

Antigen-antibody complexes: Immune complexes form when antibody binds to antigen (defined above) in the blood. The formation of the antigen-antibody complex usually involves another protein called complement. This is a factor in autoimmune disease.

Arthritis: A term commonly used to describe joint disease causing pain. It should, however, be reserved for inflammatory disease of joints, as rheumatoid arthritis.

Artificial insemination: Achieving pregnancy by artificial means; most commonly semen from a male donor is injected mechanically into the woman's vagina and or uterus.

Autoimmunity: The consequence of the arousal of the immune system leading to antibody production or a cellular (lymphocyte) reaction directed against self. The autoimmune response is an immune response generated against tissues in ones own body (antigens). This response may be antibody mediated, as a result of antigen-antibody complexes, lymphocyte mediated or both by antibody and lymphocytes.

Axon: A nerve fiber arising from a neuron (nerve cell). Signals (messages) arising from one neuron are transmitted to another via the axon.

Bacteria: Microscopic infectious organisms that cause a variety of diseases in humans and other species.

Biofeedback: A training technique that enables a patient to gain voluntary control over autonomic function.

Brain-derived nerve growth factor (BDNGF): A specific nervous system hormone which can stimulate repair of the nervous system. It was originally found in the brain but more recently it has been found that it can be produced by cell causing inflammation in the brain.

Cataracts: Any opacification (loss of transparency) of the lens or its capsule. They are not considered significant if they do not interfere with vision.

Catheterization [Bladder]: Removal of urine from the bladder by means of a urinary catheter (tube).

Cell: The smallest unit of a living animal. Cells are enclosed in a membrane (the cell membrane). They have a nucleus containing chromosomes, mitochondria and other "machinery."

Central nervous system (CNS): The term CNS refers to the brain and spinal cord.

Cerebellum: The part of the brain that controls movement, resulting in coordinated movement. It is located behind the brainstem and under the cerebral hemispheres and resembles a pair of tennis balls stuck to the brain stem.

Cervical spondylosis: A disease in which the disks between the vertebral bodies in the neck extrude like mortar between bricks. Sometimes the disks will compress the spinal cord, producing "MS-like" symptoms of weak-

ness and loss of sensation in the legs. The disease process can result in pressure on nerve roots as they leave the spinal canal, resulting in weakness and/or pain in the arms and hands.

Charcot's triad: The collection of symptoms includes nystagmus (shaky eyes), dysarthria, and tremor (slurred speech and shaking of the hands and body) that was described as being characteristic of MS. Although occurring in MS, it is rare.

Chemotherapy: Treatment with chemicals such as treatments that are used for cancer. Examples include cyclophosphamide (Cytoxan), 6-mercaptopurine, amongst others.

Chlamydia pneumoniae: A bacterium that can cause pneumonia that has been studied as a potential factor in MS as well as other diseases. It is not the organism that causes genital infections in men and women.

Chromosome: Genetic material in the nucleus within each cell is collected in structures called chromosomes. Each human female cell contains 23 pairs of homologous chromosomes: 22 pairs of autosomes, 1 pair of X chromosomes. The human male contains the same 22 pairs of autosomes but only one X chromosome with one Y chromosome.

Clinically isolated syndrome (CIS): Optic neuritis, acute vertigo or other isolated brainstem symptoms, or transverse myelitis may be referred to as CIS and may qualify for a diagnosis of MS when certain MRI abnormalities are present.

Clitoral engorgement: Blood flow to the female sexual organ, the clitoris, is associated with sexual excitement and results in clitoral enlargement (engorgement), and ultimately improves arousal and orgasm (sexual climax) in women

Cortex (cerebral cortex): The layer of neurons covering the entire outside surface of the brain. It appears gray as compared with the white matter inside the brain.

Cortisol: The primary steroid hormone (17 hydroxy-corticoid) produced by the adrenal gland. It is the biologically active soluble form of cortisone.

Cortisone: The stored form of cortisol produced by the adrenal cortex.

Cognition: Ability to reason.

Crohn's disease: An autoimmune inflammatory disease of bowel principally, but not exclusively, affecting small bowel. It occurs with increased frequency in MS patients.

Cystitis: Inflammation of the bladder associated with symptoms of urinary frequency and urgency.

Cytomegaloviruses: A family of herpes viruses that inhabit the urinary tract of almost all humans. Several subtypes have been described and appear to have geographic distributions.

Demyelinating disease: Diseases caused by demyelination. Disease primarily associated with damage to myelin, e.g. acute disseminated encephalomyelitis and MS.

Demyelination: The loss of myelin surrounding the axon, or nerve fiber, regardless of the disease process.

Dental amalgam: The material dentists used for dental repairs (make dental fillings).

Detrusor muscle: The muscle of the urinary bladder that forms the actual storage organ and is the largest part of the bladder.

Distemper: Illness in dogs and cats caused by the measles like distemper paramyxovirus of the same name.

Dysarthria: Slurred speech.

Dystonia: Abnormal muscle tone usually resulting in an abnormal position (posture) relative to the rest of the body.

EDSS (Extended Disability Status Scale): A grading scale for recording levels of neurological disability. It was originally developed by Kurtzke. It is used universally for recording disability.

Encephalomyelitis: An illness associated with inflammation of the brain and spinal cord.

Enemas: Liquids that are used to facilitate bowel evacuation; usually water or oil based materials. They are put into the rectum via an enema tube attached to a bag or other container.

Environmental factor: Any factor in the environment that may contribute to the risk of a disease, such as MS.

The environmental factor in MS is assumed to be a virus.

Epilepsy: A brain disorder that occurs when the electrical signals in the brain are disrupted leading to a seizure. Seizures can cause brief changes in a person's body movements, awareness, emotions, and senses. Some people may only have a single seizure during their lives and does not mean that a person has epilepsy. People with epilepsy have repeated seizures. Epileptic seizures eventually occur in one of ten patients with MS.

Epstein-Barr virus: The CDC definition is as follows: Epstein-Barr virus, frequently referred to as EBV, is a member of the herpesvirus family and one of the most common human viruses. The virus occurs worldwide, and most people become infected with EBV sometime during their lives. In the United States, as many as 95% of adults between 35 and 40 years of age have been infected. Infants become susceptible to EBV as soon as maternal antibody protection (present at birth) disappears. Many children become infected with EBV, and these infections usually cause no symptoms or are indistinguishable from the other mild, brief illnesses of childhood. In the United States and in other developed countries, many persons are not infected with EBV in their childhood years. When infection with EBV occurs during adolescence or young adulthood, it causes infectious mononucleosis 35% to 50% of the time.

Erectile dysfunction: The National Institutes of Health (NIH) defines erectile dysfunction as the repeated inability to get or keep an erection firm enough for sexual intercourse. The word "impotence" may also be used to describe other problems that interfere with sexual intercourse and reproduction, such as lack of sexual desire and problems with ejaculation or orgasm. Using the term erectile dysfunction makes it clear that those other problems are not involved.

Estrogen: The steroid produced by the ovary that is responsible for the secondary sexual characteristics of adult females.

Extended Disability Status Scale (EDSS): A grading scale for recording levels of neurologic disability. Kurtzke originally developed it. It is used universally for recording disability.

Familial infantile spastic paraplegia: A group of different genetic disorders that cause spasticity in family members, usually occurring in infancy. Early onset in a family setting ordinarily easily distinguishes these rare disorders from MS.

Fatigability: The loss of muscle strength following repeated use or testing of one or more muscles. In the clinical neurological examination the inability to continue walking at least 500 meters is interpreted as a meaningful degree of fatigability of the lower extremities (legs). This is used by social security for disability determinations.

Fatigue: Fatigue is different from drowsiness. Drowsiness is feeling the need to sleep, whereas fatigue is a lack of energy and motivation. Apathy (a feeling of indifference or not caring about what happens) and drowsiness can be symptoms of fatigue. Fatigue can be normal after physical exertion or because of lack of sleep. When persisting fatigue is not relieved by enough sleep, good nutrition, or a low-stress environment, it should be investigated. Because fatigue is a common complaint, associated illness may be overlooked. It is a common symptom in MS and other autoimmune disorders. However, there are many other possible physical and psychological causes of fatigue including anemia, hypothyroidism, infections, sleep disorders, depression, medications, etc. Chronic fatigue syndrome (CFS) is a condition that starts with flu-like symptoms and lasts for 6 months or more. All other possible causes of fatigue are eliminated before this diagnosis is made.

Gadolinium: An injected contrast material used to make blood vessels (or tumors) more visible on MRI brain or other tissue scans.

Gastrocnemius: The large calf muscle that pulls and keeps the foot down (plantarflexes the foot).

Gene: The smallest amount of DNA in chromosomes or mitochondria that codes for a heritable characteristic or feature.

Genetic: Any issue or consideration having to do with heredity, genes or gene changes (mutations). Also, an inherited characteristic or change.

Genital herpes: Genital herpes is a contagious viral infection primarily affecting the genitals of men and women. It is characterized by recurrent clusters of vesicles and lesions in the affected areas and is caused by the herpes simplex-2 virus (HSV-2). This virus is one of several species of the herpes virus responsible for chickenpox, shingles, mononucleosis, and oral herpes (fever blisters or cold sores, HSV-1). Infections have reached epidemic proportions with 500,000 diagnosed each year in the U.S. One in five American adults has genital herpes.

Glaucoma: The disease of the eye characterized by increased intraocular pressure causing damage to the retinal and impaired vision.

Gray matter: The cortex of the brain is the outermost layer of the brain and is made up of neurons. It completely covers the white matter. The neurons in the cortex send nerve fibers to, and receive them, from other parts of the brain and spinal cord.

Gynecologists: Physicians who specialize in diseases that uniquely affect women.

Hereditary: Transmitted from parent to child by information contained in the genes. See gene and genetics.

Herpes: Several species of the herpes viruses are responsible for disease including chickenpox, shingles, mononucleosis, oral herpes (fever blisters or cold sores, HSV-1) and roseola infantum. These are DNA viruses.

HIV: Human immunodeficiency virus, the AIDS virus.

Hormone: The internal secretion of an endocrine organ such as the adrenal or ovary. Hormones are important chemical messengers that communicate with distant organs in the body.

Hypnotism: The use of suggestion; the field of study which encompasses, among other things, hypnotic trance; its induction, management, and application; and related subjects such as the phenomena of waking suggestion. Hypnotherapy is defined as the use of therapeutic techniques or principles in conjunction with hypnosis.

Hyporeflexic bladder: Decreased bladder reactivity as defined by urodynamic testing in a laboratory.

Hypothyroidism: A disease of the thyroid associated with decreased secretion of thyroid hormone.

Immune system: The host defense against infection comprised of the white blood cells (leukocytes) including lymphocytes and monocytes circulating in the blood and other tissues (including the bone marrow), lymph nodes, and the thymus. Immunology is the study of all aspects of host defense against infection and of adverse consequences of immune responses.

Immunoglobulin: Another word for antibody.

Immunomodulation: Treatment aimed at changing immune responses to benefit a patient with autoimmune disease.

Immunosuppressive therapy: Any treatment that results in decreased immune responses. Commonly used treatments in MS that are immunosuppressive are steroids (prednisone, Medrol, Imuran, Cytoxan, and Novantrone). The interferons (Avonex, Betaseron, Rebif and Copaxone impact immune responses but are termed immunomodulatory drugs.

Immunotherapy: Treatment of any kind directed against normal or abnormal immune function, whether involving the products of the immune system or not.

Incontinence: Urinary incontinence; involuntary loss of bladder control.

Infectious mononucleosis: Glandular fever. It is a common form of infection with the Epstein-Barr virus (EBV) consisting of fever, fatigue, enlarged lymph nodes, often with rash, splenic enlargement and hepatic enzyme elevation.

Inflammation: The accumulation of fluid, plasma proteins, and white blood cells initiated by physical injury, infection, or local immune response.

Interferons: Cytokines; proteins made by lymphocytes that can induce cells to resist viral replication.

Intrathecal: Inside the central nervous system.

Lesion: Localized area of tissue damage, or pathology, regardless of cause.

Libido: Sexual interest or drive.

Lymph glands: Collections of lymphocytes into organs of immune function also called lymph nodes. They are numerous in certain parts of the body including the neck, axillae (arm pits), and groins.

Lymphocytes: Citizens of the immune system.

Macrophages: Monocytes from the blood stream that have been "turned on" by interacting with lymphocytes.

Magnetic resonance imaging (MRI): Imaging of the brain or other organs obtained by the use of magnetic fields and radio frequency together with computerized tomography.

Malignant MS: Frequent severe relapses with a rapid increase in disability constitute a very small but important subgroup of MS.

Manic psychosis: A state of elevated mood and psychosis.

Metalloproteases (MMP): Members of a group of secreted neutral proteases that degrade the collagens of the extracellular matrix. Members of this group are important in the integrity of the blood-brain barrier. MMP9 appears to be the most important of the group in this regard. MMP9 is inhibited by interferon-beta (Avonex, Betaseron, and Rebif).

Mitochondria: The cells' power sources. They usually are rod-shaped but can be round. They have an outer membrane that limits the organelle and an inner membrane thrown into folds projecting inwards i.e. "cristae mitochondriales."

Molecule: A very small mass of matter; the smallest amount of a substance which can exist alone and must consist of at least 2 atoms.

Monocytes: A leukocyte (white blood cell), they are part of the human body's immune system that protect against infections and move quickly to sites of infection. Monocytes are one of the 5 major types of white blood cells, and the name is based on their appearance in stained smears under a microscope. They are larger than red blood cells and are typically identified in laboratories by flow cytometry by their surface expression of the protein CD14. Monocytes are produced by the bone marrow from stem cell precursors, circulate in the blood stream for about one to three days and then typically move into tissues throughout the body. In the tissues monocytes mature into different types of macrophages at different anatomical locations. Monocytes which migrate from the blood stream to other tissues are called macrophages. These cells are responsible for phagocytosis, or digestion, of foreign substances in the body. An important function is the presentation of partially digested proteins via the MHC class II protein to lymphocytes T-cell receptors to initiate specific cellular immune responses, as in experimental allergic encephalomyelitis. This is thought to be important in MS, also.

MOG (myelin-oligodendrocyte glycoprotein): Specific protein found in oligodendrocytes and in myelin.

Multiple sclerosis: A neurologic disease that is characterized by focal demyelination in the central nervous system, lymphocytic infiltration in the brain, with a variably progressive course.

MRI (Magnetic resonance imaging): Imaging of the brain or other organs obtained by the use of magnetic fields and radio frequency together with computerized tomography.

Mutation: A change in the structure of DNA with a potential to alter the normal function of the gene.

Myelin: Lipoproteinaceous material composed of alternating layers of lipid and protein of the myelin sheath.

Myelin basic protein: A structural protein of myelin. It is the most antigenic protein in myelin, meaning it is the most potent protein capable of stimulating the immune system. It is highly effective in minuscule amounts in producing experimental (auto)allergic encephalomyelitis, an experimental form of MS.

Myelin oligodendrocyte glycoprotein (MOG): specific protein found in oligodendrocytes and in myelin.

Myelogram: X-ray studies of the spinal cord and spinal canal performed by the injection of contrast media. CT and MRI studies have replaced this procedure.

Myopia: Short sightedness.

Narcotics: Derived from the Greek word for stupor, that originally referred to a variety of substances that dulled the senses and relieved pain. Narcotics may be defined chemically as substances that bind at opiate receptors (cellular membrane proteins activated by substances like heroin or morphine). Some refer to any illicit substance as a narcotic. In a legal context, narcotic refers to opium, opium derivatives, and their semi-synthetic substitutes. The term narcotic is used to refer to drugs that produce morphine-like effects.

Necrosis: Tissue death; a state of irreversible tissue damage.

Neurologist: A physician specializing in the diagnosis and care of neurological disease.

Neuron: Nerve cell; the morphologic and functional unit of the nervous system. It consists of the nerve cell body, the dendrite, and the axon.

Nucleus: The cellular organelle enclosing the chromosomes. It is bounded by a nuclear membrane.

Nystagmus: fine rhythmic oscillating movements of the eyeball.

Oligoclonal band: Bands of antibody that are present on electrophoresis of CSF.

Oligodendrocyte: Glial cells that give rise to the myelin sheath. Each cell forms several myelin sheaths.

Ophthalmologists: Physicians specialized in the diagnosis and treatment of diseases of the eye.

Optic nerve: The second cranial nerve which is actually an extension of the brain. Nerve fibers from the retina travel to the brain through the optic nerves.

Optic neuritis (retrobulbar neuritis): An inflammation of the optic nerve with pain and variable loss of vision. Most patients will eventually be diagnosed as having MS.

Orgasm: Sexual climax.

Osteopenia and Osteoporosis: Osteoporosis, or porous bone, is a disease characterized by low bone mass and structural deterioration of bone tissue, leading to bone fragility and an increased risk of fractures of the hip, spine, and wrist. Men as well as women are affected by osteoporosis, a disease that can be prevented and treated. Osteopenia is a lesser degree of bone loss. Bone densitometry is an accurate way of detecting this bone loss and monitoring treatment.

Pathology: The scientific study of disease. It is also a term used to describe detectable damage to tissues.

Pituitary gland: An endocrine gland about the size of a pea at the base of the brain. Its posterior lobe is connected to a part of the brain called the hypothalamus. The anterior pituitary lobe receives releasing hormones from the hypothalamus. The pituitary gland secretes hormones regulating a wide variety of bodily activities, including trophic hormones that stimulate other endocrine glands. ACTH is but one of the hormones secreted by the pituitary and it regulates steroid production by the adrenal gland. The pituitary is regulated by releasing hormones from the hypothalamus.

Plaque: The plate-like hardened areas of myelin damage and scarring in MS located in the brain and spinal cord.

Pneumocystis: A one-cell organism that causes rapidly fatal lung infestations in AIDS patients.

Polymorphisms: Referring to genetic polymorphisms, meaning many forms or shapes indicating the presence of mutations, chromosomal breaks, and transpositions, etc.

Postinfectious encephalomyelitis: Acute disseminated encephalomyelitis occurring following an infection.

Progressive multifocal leukoencephalopathy (PML): A serious infection of the brain caused by the JC papilloma virus.

Proteolipid: A structural protein of myelin. It can be used to sensitize mice and produce a form of experimental allergic encephalomyelitis.

Pyelonephritis: An acute infection of the kidney associated with fever, contrasting with cystitis (a bladder infection) where fever does not occur.

Pyramidal tract: The nerve fiber tract in the brainstem and spinal cord comprised of the nerve fibers arising from the motor cortex.

Rapidly progressive MS: (Marburg's variant of multiple sclerosis) is a very aggressive form of MS where the disease advances quickly and relentlessly leading to rapid disability and death. It is also known as acute or fulminant MS. Marburg's MS often strikes in younger people and is often preceded by or associated with fever.

Relapse: Appearance of new signs or recurrence of previous signs of MS.

Rheumatoid arthritis: A common inflammatory joint disease caused by an autoimmune response.

Sclerotic: A term referring to hardened tissue such as MS plaques in the brain. This hardness or sclerosis is caused by scarring.

Seizure: An epileptic event consisting of loss of consciousness usually associated with tonic and/or clonic movements.

Semen: The fluid portion of the ejaculate consisting of secretions from the seminal vesicles, prostate gland, and several other glands in the male reproductive tract. Semen may also refer to the entire ejaculate, including the sperm.

Shingles: Skin infection caused by the herpes zoster virus. They are typically associated with pain.

Single nucleotide polymorphisms (SNPs): A group of gene alterations that may be a "signature group" for a disease.

Spinal fluid (CSF): Fluid produced by the choroid plexus within the brain. It is located in the ventricles and surrounds the brain and spinal cord.

Spinal MS: The older term for primary progressive MS which was commonly used prior to the modern era of imaging.

Spasticity: Velocity-dependent increase in muscle tone.

Sphincter: The sphincter is a circular muscle that constricts a passage such as the urethra or anus. When relaxed, a sphincter allows materials to pass through the opening and when contracted, it closes the opening.

Steroids: A large family of chemical substances, including many hormones, chemically defined as containing a tetracyclic cyclopenta alpha phenanthrene skeleton.

Syphilis: An infection due to *Treponema pallidum*. These infections are similar in type to infections by tuberculosis but are potentially more serious. One type (meningo-vascular syphilis) can cause small strokes and manifestations may resemble MS.

Systemic infections: As opposed to a localized infection, a system infection is any infection which causes generalized symptoms. It is usually associated with a fever. A septicemia would be an example of a severe generalized infection. "Sepsis" is a colloquial (slang) term for a systemic bacterial infection of the bloodstream. It is a very serious, frequently fatal condition. Infection with gram negative bacteria triggers septic shock via TNF-α (tissue necrosis factor alpha or lymphotoxin).

Systemic lupus erythematosus (SLE): A chronic inflammatory autoimmune disorder that may affect many organ systems including the skin, joints and internal organs. The disease may be mild or severe and life-threatening. African-Americans and Asians are disproportionately affected. The ANA test helping in the diagnosis of SLE is positive in about one half of MS patients.

T-cell: A subset of lymphocytes developing in the thymus. Killer T-cell is the common term for a cytotoxic T-cell. T-cells are thymus-dependent lymphocytes that fail to develop in the absence of a functional thymus.

T-cell growth factor beta-1: An interleukin (hormone) produced by lymphocytes that stimulates scarring in tissues. It also stimulates myelin formation.

Testosterone: The principal steroid hormone produced by the male testicles, and to a lesser extent by the adrenal cortex. It is responsible for stimulating sexual development at male adolescence. It has a positive effect on protein metabolism (an anabolic effect).

Tetanus: A potentially fatal illness produced by infection with the bacterium *Clostridium tentani* most often complicating wound contamination.

It is characterized by rapidly increasing stiffness and may lead to seizures and death.

Thrush: Throat infection by the yeast *Candida albicans.* It commonly complicates treatment with antibiotics and steroids.

Toxoplasmosis: Infestation of the human body by the one celled animal *Toxoplasma gondii.*

Transverse myelitis: signs of spinal cord damage appearing acutely or subacutely with signs of inflammation. When accompanied by certain brain MRI abnormalities, it may qualify for a diagnosis of CIS/MS.

Tremor: An oscillating rhythmic movement usually involving an extremity. Head movement may accompany tremor but is termed titubation.

Trigeminal neuralgia: Intense, brief, facial pain typically occurring on one side. It is uncommon before 65 years of age, except in MS. Its occurrence in young adults is usually a sign of MS.

Tuberculosis: The disease that results from infection by *Mycobacterium tuberculosis.* Although most commonly affecting the lungs, any tissue in the body can be involved.

Tumor necrosis factor: A principal factor made by macrophages that damage myelin.

Urethra: The anatomical tube connecting the bladder with the outside of the body. In the male it extends to the opening in the penis.

Urology: The field of medical care dealing with diseases of the kidneys, bladder, and associated structures including the ureters, urethra, etc. In men the field deals with diseases of the male generative organs, also.

Vaccination: The deliberate induction of adaptive immunity to a pathogen by injecting a vaccine, a dead or attenuated (nonpathogenic) form of the pathogen.

Virus: Pathogens composed of a nucleic acid genome enclosed in a protein coat. Viruses can replicate only in a living cell.

White blood cells: Leukocytes of the blood. A general term used for all white blood cells including lymphocytes, polymorphonuclear leukocytes and monocytes.

White matter: White matter of the brain is largely made of myelin and gets its name because it has a lot of fat in it and looks whitish compared to the cortex.

Yeast vaginitis: A common infection due to the yeast *Candida albicans*.

Index

Index